RIDGEVIEW MEDICAL

New Solutions for Joint Pain

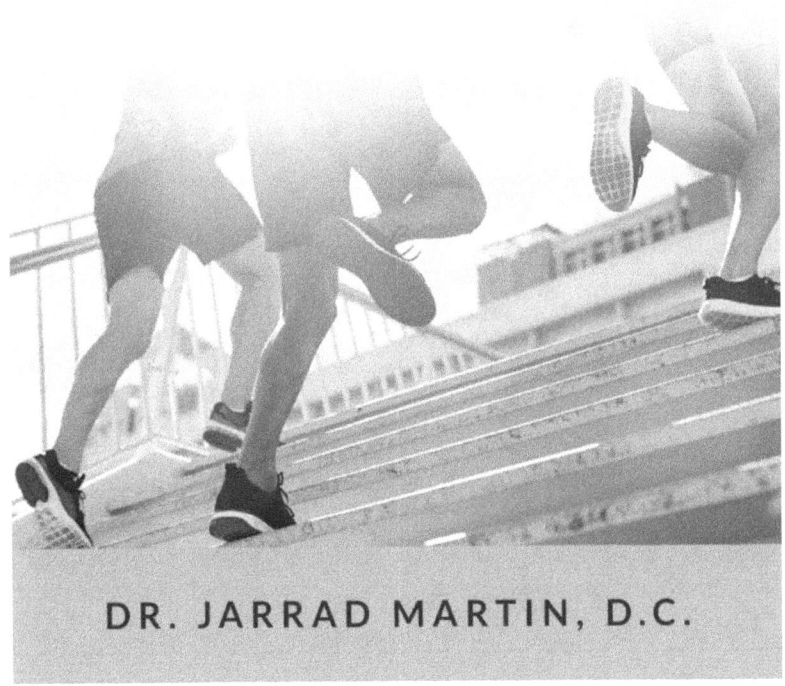

DR. JARRAD MARTIN, D.C.

Ridgeview Medical
New Solutions for Joint Pain

Taking chronic pain management to the next level

Dr. Jarrad Martin, D.C.

Ridgeview Medical
New Solutions for Joint Pain

Trademark 2021 by Ridgeview Medical

All rights reserved. Copyright under Berne Copyright Convention, Universal Copyright Convention, and Pan-American Copyright Convention. No part of this book may be reproduced, stored in a retrieval system, or transmitted in any form, or by any means, electronic, mechanical, photocopying, recording or otherwise, without prior permission of the author.

ISBN: 9798746773760

Published by Ridgeview Medical

Disclaimer

While the authors have used their best efforts in preparing this book, they make no representations or warranties with respect to accuracy or completeness of the contents of this book. The advice and strategies contained herein may not be suitable for your situation. You should consult a professional where appropriate. The authors shall not be liable for any loss of profit or any other special, incidental, consequential, or other damages. The purchaser or reader of this publication assumes responsibility for the use of these materials and information. Adherence to all applicable laws and regulations, both advertising and all other aspects of doing business in the United States or any other jurisdiction, is the sole responsibility of the purchaser or reader.

Special Thanks & Dedications

I would like to acknowledge and thank Dr's. Mike and Colleen Carberry whom without I would not have had the tools to found Ridgeview Medical as an Integrated Medical office. Bob Beilhart for implementing a business technology into these clinics. Bobbi Palmer for his street smarts. Brandon Dawson who will take us to new heights. Signature Biologics and Predictive Biotech. The Driving Force for pushing me to finally write a book.

My mother and father for infinite support.

To all my coaches through the years: Dr. Greg Lohman, Dr. Steve Hays, Dr. James Bridges, Michael Boyd, Shervon Lakeberg, Dr. Joe Dziezgowski, Leslie Berneske, Robb Henderson, Octavio Mella, Kelly Hudson, Dr. Karl Jawhari, Dr. James Fowler, Rachel Black and George "Force" Chamberlain for helping me stay on track and confront the impossible.

Attorney Josh Massengill for having Chiropractor's backs in Texas.

Kasey Grounds, one of the most awesome people walking the planet that I am privileged to have on my team and who I would not have been able to integrate without.

Dr. Fabrizio Mancini and Jack Canfield for inspiration.

Tim Holcomb FNP-C and Ismail Salejee, MD.

Grant Cardone. The man who's books that changed my life forever.

Table of Contents

SPECIAL THANKS & DEDICATIONS 4

CHAPTER 1 7
   Dr. Jarrad Martin, D.C. & Ridgeview Medical 7

CHAPTER 2 13
   Skeletal Alignment 13

CHAPTER 3 21
   Regenerative Medicine 21

CHAPTER 4 35
   PRP 35

CHAPTER 5 41
   Bracing 41

CHAPTER 6 49
   Knee Pain 49

CHAPTER 7 53
   Low Back Pain 53

CHAPTER 8 61
   Physiotherapy and Rehab 61

CHAPTER 9 65
   Sciatica 65

CHAPTER 10 69
   Trigger Point Injections 69

CHAPTER 11 73
   What Patients Are Saying 73

CHAPTER 12 81
   Supportive Studies 81

Chapter 1

Dr. Jarrad Martin, D.C. & Ridgeview Medical

About Dr. Jarrad Martin, D.C.

Dr. Martin spent 8 years working in the pharmaceutical industry where he became increasingly frustrated by the lack of true healing patients were experiencing by treating their symptoms with medication. He departed from a career in pharmaceuticals to find solutions that focused on the CAUSE of a patient's problem, rather than just treating the SYMPTOMS.

On his journey to find a new perspective on healing, Dr. Martin found his place at the Harvard of Chiropractic Schools, Parker University. At Parker, Dr. Martin dedicated years to learning about how true healing comes through proper skeletal alignment, functional improvement, modification of the typical American lifestyle, and reduction in the daily poisons that come with it.

After over 7 years of successfully treating patients with chronic pain from degenerative arthritis, Dr. Martin founded Ridgeview Medical. Ridgeview Medical is an integrated medical clinic that utilizes a multidisciplinary team approach to patient care. This way Ridgeview Medical can offer an array of diagnostic and treatment options, from multiple healthcare practitioners, all under one roof. Ridgeview Medical is also one of the only Medical Clinics in the North Texas area providing regenerative therapy.

Dr. Martin has been a licensed Chiropractor serving the North Dallas community since graduating from Parker University in 2013.

Ridgeview Medical

About 56 Million Americans today suffer from the effects of chronic pain. That's about 20% of all the adults in the United States, and the numbers continue to rise. If you are experiencing chronic pain brought on by stress, medical conditions, or even from an accident, our friendly staff is ready to help you by bringing you the most cutting-edge treatments and therapies.

What's unfortunate for most people is that their pain could be relieved. They just don't know where to turn for help and many unfortunate people go untreated until surgery is the only option left. Ridgeview Medical is dedicated to helping you not only relieve your pain, but restore your function. We offer the best approach to pain relief and injury recovery through non-opioid, non-surgical approaches. We are committed to providing you with the best in health care techniques and technologies for an individualized approach to your health and well-being. We want to help you get your life back.

Do you suffer from chronic pain?

The truth today is that the majority of chronic pain patients can be helped. The difficulty is finding a provider that does not blindly follow the typical outdated treatment cycle of drugs (including opioids), cortisone shots, arthroscopy and then replacement or fusion surgery. According to overdosefreeamerica.org, opioids are the leading cause of death for Americans under 50 yoa and over 527,000 prescriptions are written daily for opioids. That's right, daily. Moreover, opioids only mask the pain while the problem is almost always getting worse. Our clinic offers completely different approach. We have multiple options available to fit the many different problems that exist. Our goal is get you off of long-term pain medications and avoid the surgery you may have been told you need.

We offer services such as Regenerative Medicine, Platelet-Rich Plasma, Hyaluronic Acid Injections, Trigger Point Injections, Chiropractic and Rehabilitative Exercises, Back Bracing, Knee Bracing, Orthotics, TENS, Functional Re-Exams, Re-xrays and Individualized Comprehensive Careplans.

Why our approach is different?

At Ridgeview Medical we offer an array of services not found in most healthcare settings. Our ability to offer the best in medical and alternative treatments in one location means that our patients have more options. Our team will work with you to develop a treatment plan that makes sense for you.

Make today be the day that you change your life and your health. Schedule a free consultation today with our team so that we can get a better understanding of your needs. We will work with you one on one to help you overcome the pain you are experiencing.

Are you tired of feeling the way you're feeling? At Ridgeview Medical our team is ready to meet with you to discuss your needs. We will help to design a program that is right for you. We look forward to meeting you.

Chapter 2

Skeletal Alignment

What is skeletal alignment?

If you were watering your lawn with a water-hose and suddenly the water stopped, how much time would you spend investigating the end of the hose where the water comes out? Almost no time right, because you know the problem is not where the water was coming out (the symptom). You know somewhere else there is a kink in the hose. The body is the same way. The CAUSE of the problem may not be where the symptom presents. The body adapts to pain by over-utilizing another area.

For this reason, it is always important to check, not only the other knee but the alignment of their entire skeleton. Often times, in the past at some point, the asymptomatic knee gave them trouble and they adapted by favoring the symptomatic knee. Our body has an amazing ability to adapt. Finding out the CAUSE of why they are having knee pain in the first place is paramount. This is why it is always important to check the other knee as well as the alignment of their spine and pelvis. Gravity is always pushing straight down on us. If the alignment of our skeleton looks like the leaning tower of Pisa . . . it must be corrected to take undue pressure off the joints. Knee pain can be caused by misalignments of the spine all the way up to the neck and shoulders, however, let's consider just the pelvis for example. If the pelvis is misaligned a non-anatomical short leg is created. Although subtle, a slightly short leg due to pelvic misalignment can put undue strain on the knees. If skeletal misalignment is not evaluated, and only the symptomatic knee is treated, the body will just find another joint to wear out.

How do you treat for this?

We utilize a proprietary method to correct and align the skeleton. Currently, the best way to check alignment is with an x-ray. In our office we take a digital x-ray of the spine, pelvis and knees. Then we analyze the x-rays by drawing vertical and horizontal lines to see if there is in fact a skeletal misalignment. If there is, it must be addressed to fully correct the cause of the knee pain. A treatment plan is created by our team of doctors which includes corrective rehabilitative exercises (for the muscles, tendons and ligaments) and chiropractic (to align the spine and pelvis). The corrective rehab includes Pettibon neck traction to restore spinal motion and reduce pain through repetitive loading and unloading of the cervical and thoracic spine. By pumping fluid in and waste out, they deliver much needed nutrients to white tissues, rehydrating and restoring disc height. This process helps to restore normal spinal curves and accelerates successful rehab. Balance discs are used specifically to provide often much needed flexibility and rehydration to the discs of the lumbar spine with expansion and contraction exercises. Whole body vibration (WBV) is utilized by having our patients do their corrective exercises while standing on a vibration plate. WBV therapy has a myriad of benefits. Some of these include:

- Correction of cervical curve
- Improved range of motion
- Improved posture, coordination and balance
- Reduced scoliosis
- Improved spinal stability
- Increased bone density
- Improved pelvic floor function
- Relief from menopausal symptoms
- relief from chronic pain
- Reduction in pain and inflammation due to bone loss and arthritis
- Increased hormonal production
- Increased cell oxygenation
- Improved circulation

- A reduction in cellulite
- Tightened facial muscles
- Increased libido and energy
- Increased immune function
- Increased muscle strength and tone
- Faster body detoxification

Lastly, after all the muscles and ligaments are warmed up from the initial rehab, corrective chiropractic adjustments are performed to help to realign the entire spine, balance the pelvis and uneven legs to take pressure off the knees with manual decompression and knee joint adjustments. In addition, some stretching, exercises, and spinal molding rolls may be prescribed for homework. This proprietary method ensures the fastest and most effective results for our patients.

How do patients feel after this treatment?

The best part is that our patients appreciate our whole-body approach at correcting the CAUSE of their knee pain. I never get tired of hearing how different we are than anywhere else they have gone for chronic pain. When patients experience our skeletal alignment methods, they feel so much looser and flexible. Function improves and in most cases people are able to resume activity without pain. Since the rehab is performed at the patient's own comfort level, soreness is minimized and patients usually report feeling better after the first treatment.

What is the most common question you get asked about that treatment?

My experience is that patients increasingly want to know "why" they are prescribed a certain procedure or treatment. They want to understand. Gone are the days when a patient would take the doctor's word for it. Taking the time to educate our patients about why a treatment is necessary is paramount to having an office filled with happy patients committed to getting out of pain and referring their friends and family.

What question SHOULD someone ask you about this treatment?

In truth, patients should be asking more questions. Even when taking something as widely accepted as Ibuprofen. Most people know now that Ibuprofen and Advil can have negative consequences for the digestive system. What most patients don't know is that the most recent medical studies are finding that this class of drugs (NSAIDS, or non-steroidal anti-inflammatory drugs) can destroy cartilage. Type in "NSAIDS destroy cartilage" into google and read for yourself. Scary stuff. This means the patients taking NSAIDS for joint pain may be fast tracking that joint into degeneration. One of the most common treatments for joint pain is cortisone shots. Only 4 cortisone shots in a lifetime to any one joint is recommended. As you will see in the coming chapters, there are much better alternatives now available.

What is the biggest misconception about the treatment? Often patients come in and think that one treatment will fix all their problems. I don't know where this misconception came from. Is it possible that one treatment will get rid of their pain? Absolutely! But if the underlying cause of the pain is not addressed properly, the patient will often time resume the same pain cycle in the future. That would be the equivalent of discontinuing an antibiotic before the prescribed course of treatment. We all know that the infection will most likely come back and it will be worse the second time. Therefore, completing a treatment plan that is recommended is very important. The biggest misconception about proper rehabilitation of a joint is that it has to be expensive and done by a state of the art machinery. Rehab, when done correctly, is low tech and inexpensive.

Chapter 3

Regenerative Medicine

What is regenerative medicine?

Chronic degenerative arthritis (CDA) is the number one reason for an adult to end up in the hospital. Over 90% of Americans suffer from CDA. Which means the pain or lack of being able to function in their joints has caused them to visit the hospital. One of the reasons that regenerative medicine is so exciting is the theory that certain cells injected into a degenerating joint could help the joint to regenerate.

Let's take a moment to demystify arthritis. First of all, arthritis just means "joint inflammation", in Latin. 'Arthros' means joint, and 'itis 'means inflammation. But why is the joint inflamed in the first place? The tissues on the outside of a joint inflame because the joint is not getting enough nutrition on the inside.

Healing inside of a joint is different than everywhere else in the body. Most of the body gets nutrition through blood supply. If you cut your finger, the nerves tell you something is wrong by sensing pain, and blood supply brings nutrition and healing. This is fast and efficient. A joint like the knee joint is a pressurized capsule. There is no blood supply in or out of the knee. So how does this sequestered joint capsule get nutrition in and waste products out?

If you notice in the picture below, the two bones are not touching, but in addition, the cartilage (the blue area) is

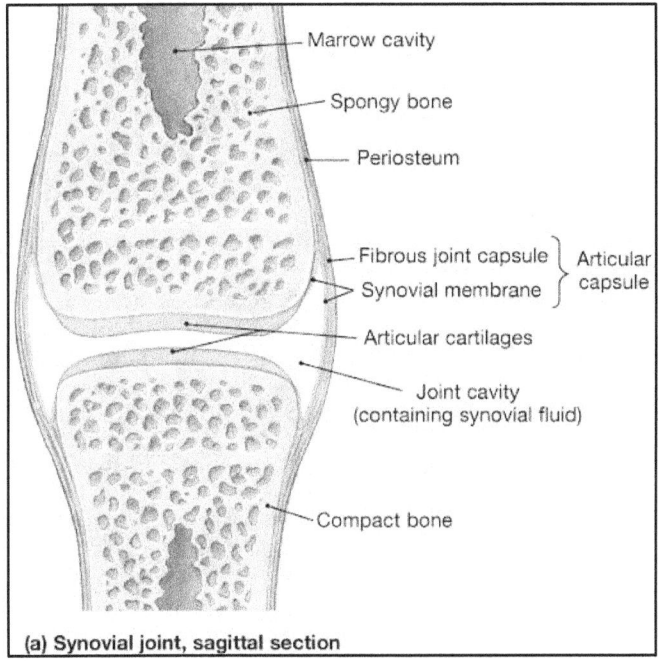

(a) Synovial joint, sagittal section

not touching either. This is because there is so much synovial fluid packed inside the joint capsule (cavity) to help lubricate the joint that nothing is touching. Your knee bones literally float on this pressurized capsule. The innate wisdom of the body knows it would be much too painful to walk around just on cartilage all the time. So how does nutrition get into the knee and waste get out? Through osmosis, assisted by the pumping motion of the knee. The outside barrier of the joint capsule allows a flow of particles inside and outside the joint with different changes in pressure inside the joint. In other words, the knee stays healthy through proper movement. As you move your knee it pumps nutrition in and toxins out.

If you do anything to restrict the movement of that joint. That joint is going to have less nutrition. When there is less nutrition, the body will try to force nutrition into the joint "Arthro" causing inflammation "itis" of the surrounding tissue. What limits the motion is scar tissue. Injuries cause microtears to the tissues. Microtears are healed by scar tissue which is less flexible than regular tissue. Arthritis shows up in areas of previous injury. Every other joint in the body has this same potential problem, including spinal joints of the low back and neck.

There is a typical standard of care that we follow in the U.S. for chronic degenerative arthritis. First, NSAIDS are prescribed, then stronger NSAIDS, opioids, then cortisone shots, then arthroscopic surgery, then full joint replacement (or fusion if in the spine). But now there is a completely new option available: regenerative medicine.

There is a regenerative revolution going on in the U.S. In my opinion, it is going to change healthcare. It already is having an enormous impact on patients lives for the better, with minimal side effects when sourced properly. I feel privileged to be able to take advantage of this new wave of unbelievable clinical results we are seeing in our clinic as well as our sister clinics across the U.S. I am part of a growing national team of medical doctors, nurse practitioners, physical therapists and Chiropractors through an amazing company called AMI (Advanced Medical Integration), who are all at the forefront of this revolution.

There are many different types and sources of regenerative medicine. What I am referring to in this book are HCTP's (Human Cellular Tissue Products). These cells include hyaluronic acid, growth hormones, cytokines, and stem cells. Lately there have been some options that have made it extremely convenient, fast, and cost effective for patients.

Stem cells are like baby cells that don't know what they want to be when they grow up. Stem cells can potentially grow into muscle cells, skin cells, bone cells, tendon cells, organ cells, nerve cells, etc. This is why stem cells are in the spot light. Specifically, mesenchymal cells are the stem cells in which scientists are focusing. Mesenchymal cells seem to be the best suited for tissue repair. The highest concentration of mesenchymal cells in the human body is in Wharton's Jelly. Wharton's Jelly is the tissue surrounding the blood vessels in the umbilical cord.

A quick note before moving forward.

A few years ago, regenerative medicine received some bad press. In fact, it was illegal to use stem cells in the U.S. until the past few years. This was in regard to stem cells from aborted fetuses. To be clear, we do NOT use embryological stem cells. No babies are sacrificed for the tissues we inject into our patients. Our HCTP's come from reputable labs that exceed industry requirements for their procedures. These placental tissues and fluid are processed in a clean room environment that exceeds AATB (American Association of Tissue Banks) standards and cleared by the FDA. Currently, there are only two labs that meet the standards to be a vendor for the AMI team of Doctors.

Signature Biologics https://www.signaturebiologics.com and Predictive Biotech https://www.predictivebiotech.com . Predictive Biotech is one of the largest regenerative medicine tissue providers and has had over 120,000 tissues injected by practitioners. Signature Biologics has recently received Investigational New Drug (IND) Approval from the FDA for Phase 1 Study in patients with symptomatic osteoarthritis of the knee. This is how Dan Wagner, Sr. Director of Business Development for Signature Biologics, describes where their tissue comes from:

"Signature Biologics only uses tissue that meets our rigorous selection criteria. Donors are health women, pre-screened by a licensed physician. Tissue is collected after a full-term live birth by c-section, conducted by licensed professionals. The C-section birth is an important component as it allows for the tissue to be collected in a controlled environment without exposure to potential contaminants that it may come in contact with otherwise."

Some History

There is research about placental tissue being used for healing for over 100 years. In 1913 in the JAMA (Journal of the American Medical Association) Dr. Maximillian Stern wrote an article called "The grafting of Preserved Amniotic Membrane to Burned and Ulcerative Surfaces, Substituting Skin Grafts". Dr. Stern was a medical doctor working in a burn unit in a hospital. One day he actually used a placenta from the birth unit to heal one of his burn patients. He essentially draped amniotic tissue over the surface of a burn and documented the burned skin healing much better than the traditionally treated burn tissue. With enough research he argued might avoid the need for grafting skin from another area of the same person's body.

Immune privileged

We have the highest concentration of stem cells in our body when we are a baby. As we get older the number of stem cells decrease. This is why babies heal so fast and we heal slower as we get older. So, the best place to harvest HCTP's ethically is from umbilical and amniotic sources.

These tissues have been found to have virtually no side effects is because these tissues are what is called "immune privileged" meaning they have DNA that is not coded to the mother or the baby. They contain a 3rd DNA that is immune privileged. This means that the innate intelligence of your body will not react to these tissues as a foreign tissue but, in theory, should instead, use them for healing when injected into the injured area. The reason this is theory is that it has not been proven. I believe it hasn't been proven yet because there is a lack of studies. In our clinic as well as our AMI sister clinics, we observe clinical improvements in our patients. The U.S. is now ramping up regenerative medicine studies, however, the truth is our healthcare system is geared toward pharmaceuticals and surgical procedures and that is where most of the resources are allocated. Over the past few years, the reason that HCTP's are in the spotlight is because other countries have been pulling back the veil. Change has been slow but, in my opinion, regenerative medicine is about to skyrocket into public view. The demand for these tissues is already high and the reason the tissues can be expensive to obtain as they can't always predict when the mother is going to have her baby and they have to be at the ready with their clean room procedures. I have included multiple studies at the end of this book.

Cost

In the past stem cell treatments were very lengthy and could cost tens of thousands of dollars. This is because it included possibly harvesting a person's own HCTP's by using adipose (fat) tissue or bone marrow to get stem cells and inject it back into the patient. Often times they would not find enough cells and have to ship them outside of the U.S. to another country where it was legal to grow the stem cells. In that case it could be tens of thousands of dollars. Today, by utilizing HCTP's from amniotic and umbilical sources the procedures generally cost anywhere from $5,000 to $11,000 per mL. Usually, 1mL is needed per joint. Compared to the alternatives of ineffectiveness of damage from drugs and dangers of surgery, in my opinion this is a no brainer.

How do you treat for this?

This is a 10-minute procedure in our clinic. First a patient is evaluated by our medical team as a candidate for regenerative medicine and educated about the procedure. The Nurse Practitioner will prep the area with alcohol and/or iodine swab. Lidocaine or a cold spray may be used to numb the area of injection. Ultrasound is often utilized to view inside the joint or even used as a guide while injecting the HCTP's. A small needle is inserted into the joint, the HCTP's are injected and a Band-Aid applied. There is no Anesthesia, no hospital stays, and no antibiotics.

How do patients feel after this treatment?

After the injection is performed, the patient stands up and walks out of the clinic. There is no downtime. There is no burning sensation associated with steroid injections. The only reports have been sometimes some slight local swelling, injection site ache, or light fever, which all subside within hours. Nothing has been life threatening; nothing has been long-lasting. There is no comparison to surgery for the time, downtime, rehab after surgery or cost. Clinically we expect significant improved function in 1-3 months. Everyone of course is different, but these tissues need some time to heal.

What is the most common question you get asked about this treatment?

Most commonly patients have questions about research. I have included many studies at the end of this book. However, most of the time patients just want to look at all their options. When it comes to joint pain there are not infinite options. And unlike regenerative medicine, no other procedure has the chance to potentially regenerate much needed tissue. Medications and cortisone shots mask the symptoms while the compromised joint continues to degenerate. Both are suspect of accelerating the damage. More Imaging, although helpful for diagnosis is not a treatment and often postpones much needed treatment. Arthroscopic surgery to "clean up the joint" may buy some time but creates more scar tissue. More scar tissue means less nutrition as discussed earlier so it will always make the joint worse in the long run. I have found that no patient wants a full joint replacement, unless insurance will pay for it. Handing over responsibility for your health to an insurance company can be disastrous. Most people have already waited too long by the time they walk in my office. This again is why we educate as much as possible so a patient can feel comfortable making an informed decision and take action.

What is the biggest misconception about this treatment?

The biggest misconception about getting HCTP's is that it will have immediate results. This is why it is a terrible idea to wait until the pain is extreme or you are bone on bone. Regenerative therapy will always work better earlier once a joint is compromised. As stated above, healing can take some time. In my opinion, due to the lower cost, lack of side effects, and clinical cases we have seen in our office as well as other AMI offices, regenerative medicine is always a route to consider. Any good surgeon will tell you surgery is a last resort after all other paths are exhausted.

Chapter 4

PRP

What is Platelet-Rich Plasma?

Platelet-Rich Plasma has been made popular by many top athletes like Tiger Woods, to recover from injuries. Here is a list of some:

- Carlos Martinez – St. Louis Cardinals (MLB) Pitcher - Right shoulder injury
- Griffin Canning – Los Angeles Angels (MLB) Pitcher - Ulnar collateral ligament changes and elbow joint irritation
- Kristaps Porzingis – Dallas Mavericks (NBA) Center - Right knee soreness
- Richaun Holmes – Sacramento Kings (NBA) Power Forward - Right shoulder labral tear
- Dee Ford – San Francisco 49ers (NFL) Defensive end - Knee tendinitis
- Blaine Hardy – Detroit Tigers (MLB) Pitcher - Left elbow injury pain from partially torn flexor tendon
- Miles Mikolas – St. Louis Cardinals (MLB) Pitcher - Flexor tendon strain in right forearm
- Allie Ostrander – Boise State Distance Runner - Achilles injury

PRP is a form of regenerative medicine that uses your own HCTP's to concentrate healing in a specific area. As discussed before, we have all of these cell factors inside of us: growth factors, cytokines, stem cells. Platelets are the minuscule blood cells that are your body's first defense against injury. When you experience an injury, your body's immediate immune response signals to these platelets the need to go to the site of the injury and activate healing. PRP can help you overcome injuries to the hips, elbows, shoulders, knees, as well as specific issues such as problematic tendons and ligaments. According to Webmd, PRP injections are used to treat torn tendons, tendinitis, muscle injuries, arthritis-related pain, and joint injuries.

How do you treat for this?

PRP in our office is a 30-minute procedure. First, a vial of blood is drawn from the patient. The blood is then spun down in a centrifuge to separate the Platelet-rich Plasma from the rest of the blood. Next the Nurse Practitioner will draw the PRP into a syringe and inject it directly into the area of injury or degeneration. Lidocaine, again, may be used prior to numb the area.

As discussed earlier with regenerative medicine, the age of the HCTP's appears to play a role. The clinical cases seem to suggest that after about 40 yoa, PRP alone is not as effective as the amniotic and umbilical tissues. Our clinics will often use PRP as boosters to provide support for amniotic and umbilical tissues a month after HCTP's. This seems to kick healing into high gear.

How do patients feel after this treatment?

Patients usually feel better than they have in years after this treatment. However, this is a procedure in which the body needs time to respond to achieve that level of being pain-free or having symptoms reduced.

What is the most common question you get asked about this treatment?

Patients ask if PRP is covered on insurance. Insurance often will often not cover any type of regenerative medicine, however we can always verify when they come in the office.

What question SHOULD your patients ask you about this treatment?

Patients should instead be asking what their options are. Again, options are limited and nothing else other than regenerative medicine has the hope of regenerating a degenerating joint.

Chapter 5

Bracing

What is bracing?

Bracing can be an extremely excellent form of immediate non-narcotic pain care for knee and low back pain. The types of braces I am referring to are far from something you would buy at your local CVS or find on Amazon.

Offloading Knee Brace

Offloading knee braces are specifically designed to unload and take pressure off a knee with CDA or OA (Osteoarthritis). Most knees degenerate either on the inside of the knee (varus) or the outside of the knee (valgus). These braces, when fitted, will put pressure at key points on the joint to push it back into a normal position. These braces can help slow the degenerative process and actually buy patients some time until they can get another form of therapy. Many of our clinics now use the unloading knee braces in conjunction with HCTP injections. After the injection, the braces are worn to normalize the joint while it allows to heal.

A recent study in the British Medical Journal showed the unloader knee brace can delay surgery and indeed deem it unnecessary over the long term for patients (39%) with unicompartmental (either the inside of the knee or the outside of the knee) arthritis.

"The unloader knee brace can delay surgery and indeed deem it unnecessary over the long term for patients (39%) with unicompartmental arthritis. Patients were able to return to their daily activities and work while using the unloader knee brace. The duration of wear was proportional to a successful outcome; we recommend education, motivation and support up to 24 months to increase compliance with its use. The unloader knee brace proposes a cost-effective non-operative option for the treatment of unicompartmental knee osteoarthritis that can be quickly administered and significantly improve the patient's quality of life. Given that patients can self-select surgical intervention, the unloader knee brace has been shown to be cost-effective as either a complement, or alternative, to surgery. It is particularly useful in the younger age group (<50), as delaying surgical intervention could reduce the demand for highly complex and expensive revision knee surgery in the future."

Unloading knee braces are definitely a viable and cost-effective option for people seeking quick relief and some very promising long-term effects.

LSO Back Braces

Often with back pain the muscles in the low back go into overdrive and even though have good intention can go through a cycle of pain and spasm. With most back braces there is one wrap that provides support. LSO Back Braces, specifically from Azon Medical, have a pulley system throughout the brace that actually helps to decompress the lumbar spine, and assist the muscles into relaxing. The pulley system included within an LSO back brace creates a resistive force on low back load to decrease such load, allowing the muscles to relax and the trunk to be supported.

There are multiple reasons clinics are incorporating LSO back braces into care plans for patients with low back problems:

One major reason is to assist a patient with managing their pain at home during the duration of care-- and to decrease the dependence on Tylenol or Advil.

Patients who are given an effective tool for pain management by their doctor are less likely to seek out a harmful solution to provide them with relief.

More than 191 million opioid prescriptions were dispensed to American patients in 2017. 66% of these prescriptions were for conditions often associated with pain (most commonly, back pain).

A study conducted in 2015 showed that the #1 source for misused pain relievers was obtained from a friend or relative. The vast majority of which were provided to the user for free or taken without permission.

How do you treat for this?

These braces are stocked in our office from Azon Medical and are generally given on the first or second visit to help with pain in the knees and low back.

How do patients feel after this treatment?

I have seen first-hand the relief a patients experience with these braces. With the back braces I have noticed about a 30 second delay. I will help a patient put on the brace and invariably they will be talking and at some point, their face will change and say, "ahhh, I just felt the muscles in my lower back relax!" It makes me smile every time.

What is the most common question you get asked about this treatment?

Mostly the question with the braces is, "Will it create a dependency?" or "will it make the muscles weaker in the area if I wear it too long?". The newest studies show that this is not as much a factor when wearing these braces.

For the unloading knee brace a recent article by By Cheryl L. Hubley-Kozey, PhD, and Gillian Hatfield Murdock, PT, MSc found:

"Dose-response research refutes the common perception that increasing brace wear time leads to muscle atrophy in patients with knee osteoarthritis. In fact, longer bracing duration appears to improve hamstring strength as well as increasing patients 'physical activity levels."

Wearing a back brace all day every day obviously could become a problem. Bracing is not the end treatment but assists a patient's pain levels while offering support so a patient can begin other treatment such as core strengthening or regenerative medicine.

What question SHOULD patients ask you about this treatment?

A patient should be asking what they can do to not have to use the brace anymore.

Chapter 6

Knee Pain

Experiencing knee pain?

Knee pain can be caused by a sudden injury, an overuse injury, or by an underlying condition, such as arthritis. Treatment will vary depending on the cause. Symptoms of knee injury can include pain, swelling, and stiffness

Knee pain is an extremely common complaint, and there are many causes. It is important to make an accurate diagnosis of the cause of your symptoms so that appropriate treatment can be directed at the cause. If you suffer from knee pain call our team today. Our team can offer you some of the latest treatments available to help you overcome this painful problem.

Common knee pain causes

Arthritis - Arthritis is among the most common causes of knee pain, and there are many treatments available.

Ligament Injuries - Ligament injuries commonly occur during athletic activities and can cause discomfort and instability.

- Anterior Cruciate Ligament (ACL) Injury
- Posterior Cruciate Ligament (PCL) Injury

- Medial Collateral Ligament (MCL) Injury

Cartilage Injuries | Meniscal Tear - Cartilage tears are seen in young and old patients alike and are also an extremely common cause of knee pain.

Patellar Tendonitis - Tendonitis around the joint is most commonly of the patellar tendon, the large tendon over the front of the knee.

Chondromalacia Patella - Chondromalacia causes knee pain under the kneecap and is due to softening of the cartilage. It is most common in younger patients (15-35 years old).

Dislocating Kneecap - A dislocating kneecap causes acute symptoms during the dislocation but can also lead to chronic knee pain.

Baker's Cyst - A Baker's cyst is swelling in the back of the joint and is usually a sign of another underlying problem such as a meniscus tear.

Bursitis - The most common bursa affected around the joint is just above the kneecap. This is most common in people who kneel for work, such as gardeners or carpet layers.

Plica Syndrome - Plica syndrome is an uncommon cause of knee pain and can be difficult to diagnose. The diagnosis is usually made at the time of arthroscopy.

Osgood-Schlatter Disease - Osgood-Schlatter disease is a condition seen in adolescents and is due to irritation of the growth plate just at the front of the joint.

Osteochondritis Dissecans - Osteochondritis dissecans (OCD) is another condition seen in adolescents due to the growth of the bone around the joint.

Gout - Gout is an uncommon cause of knee pain. However, in patients who have a diagnosis of gout, it must be considered as a cause for new-onset knee pain.

Chapter 7

Low Back Pain

Experiencing low back pain?

Low back pain is a problem that many people deal with. What's even more discouraging to us is that many people have never tried the services we offer. We are here to help you know what options you may have.

If you are like many Americans, you are currently experiencing low back pain. This pain can be in your lower, middle, or upper back. An estimated 32 million Americans are suffering from low back pain at this moment and about 80% will experience it at some point in their life. Statistics such as these explain why the United States' number one cause of disability today is low back pain. This brings up many questions about low back pain causes, prevention, and treatment.

The causes of low back pain are virtually endless. The complex system of the back and spine require it to be both rigid, to support the body, as well as fluid to allow movement. This system is made up of many parts; ligaments, tendons, discs muscles, and bones are the main components that can be damaged and cause pain. While small irritations and stresses can create low back pain, it can be a result of major traumas, such as auto accidents. Because of this, it is often hard to pinpoint the exact cause of the pain.

Besides physical causes, conditions such as arthritis, obesity, urinary tract infections, and kidney stones can produce signs of lower back pain. With all of the possibilities in mind, it is important to find a doctor who is well versed in the area of pain management as well as all aspects of health, in order to correctly narrow down and find the root of the pain. Luckily, the staff at Ridgeview Medical are exactly these people. They have many years of experience and education with back pain and can accurately diagnose the problem. If this diagnosis is lacking, the smallest irritation can become overwhelming pain.

Disc bulges or herniation

In many cases, a bulging or herniated disc is the most painful cause of back pain. It is also one of the most common ones. However, it should be noted that these conditions don't always result in pain. Research has shown, through MRI use, that up to 37% of the American population has some severity of a disc bulge or herniation, many of which experience no pain. Nonetheless, the people who do experience pain from these conditions explain it to be intense and severe.

The position and type of herniation affect the type of pain felt. When the disc is misaligned, swollen, or irritated, it is possible for it to pinch a nerve, causing sharp pain and possible numbness, tingling, and weakness to the legs. Pain from this is often described as shooting and stabbing. To understand herniated discs, it helps to picture them as jelly-filled doughnuts. When the outer layer of the doughnut (discs) experiences wear and tear, they are likely to rupture and tear over time. As a result of this, the jelly can ooze out. Reversing this damage can be extremely difficult. However, the services we offer can result in the prevention of advancement in the herniation and relieve some or all of the pain.

Subluxations

While disc herniations are the most common cause of back pain, subluxations are the most overlooked. A subluxation is a medical term that describes a vertebrae in the spine that is out of place. Resulting from subluxations, normal, fluid movement is impaired and a multitude of other conditions, including pain, can prevail. Subluxations can be caused by almost anything and be almost anywhere on your spinal column.

Subluxations can be an outcome of many events such as stress, physical trauma, and toxins. In the same way that stress partially leads to ulcers in the gut, physiological bodily changes also may occur for the same reasons, displacing a vertebrae. As with most injuries, timing is vital, and the Doctors at Ridgeview Medical are experienced in locating and fixing the subluxation quickly and effectively.

Muscular sprains and tendon or ligament strains

When you partake in activities that your body is not accustomed to, sprains and strains are likely to occur. An example of this is a runner attempting to run a marathon as the first race of the summer, without training much during the winter and spring. The use of these muscles is irregular and odd for the body and the muscles, tendons, and ligaments get overworked, causing damage. Sprains of ligaments occur when the ligament is pushed past its capabilities and tears slightly. Sprains of muscles is the result of the body moving awkwardly quickly, as well as lifting heavy objects. Sprains and strains can be incredibly painful and often appear with bruising and swelling. These forms of injury are directly related to the spine, meaning medical care is able to help. We are fully capable and equipped to provide care for these types of injuries.

Stress and low back pain

Constant stresses create a vastly different physiological profile for a person than those who do not encounter these stresses. While your body is stressed, many different hormones are released to try and deal with the situation. These hormones result in increased heart rate, raised blood pressure, a changed immune system, and lowered bone density and muscle mass. When these hormones are released in the body, issues with relation to heart and digestive health, obesity, depression, and even back pain are common. When the stress hormones are released, the muscles in your body tense creating "trigger points". These points are very painful, however, can be treated with medical care.

By going after the causes of low back pain, rather than the symptoms, the results are much more successful, and the treatment becomes easier. One thing all of the conditions listed above have in common is spinal misalignment. Luckily, the expert staff at Ridgeview Medical is equipped with the knowledge and tools to work towards bettering this issue.

Like with any pain or condition, a non-invasive and conservative yet effective approach is always the first option in treating back pain. If there are any other questions you have about your condition or about low back pain as a whole, contact us at Ridgeview Medical. And if you are ready to take the leap towards health, call today and schedule an appointment.

Chapter 8

Physiotherapy and Rehab

Physiotherapy and rehab help restore function, improve mobility, relieve pain, and prevent or limit permanent physical disabilities of patients suffering from injuries or disease. Physiotherapy or "medically directed rehab" helps restore, maintain, and promote overall fitness and health. Our patients include accident victims and individuals with disabling conditions such as low-back pain, arthritis, athletic injuries and failed surgeries.

Treatment often includes exercise; especially for patients who have been immobilized or who lack flexibility, strength, or endurance. Physiotherapy helps encourage patients to use their muscles to increase their flexibility and range of motion. More advanced exercises focus on improving strength, balance, coordination, and endurance. The goal is to improve how an individual functions at work and at home. Physiotherapy also helps treat a wide range of disorders, such as pediatrics, geriatrics, orthopedics, sports medicine, neurology, and cardiopulmonary physiotherapy.

How physiotherapy and rehab works.
Ridgeview Medical was designed to provide an ideal environment for healing your body, through chiropractic, stretching and strengthening exercises, balance cushions,

orthotics and individualized comprehensive careplans.. When you arrive at our office, our Nurse Practitioner and Case Manager will take a thorough history, and evaluation of the entire body including posture and biomechanics, range of motion, and joint mobility to find out the cause of pain or disability. You will then discuss treatment options and goals so that we can customize a treatment plan catered to you.

Each session will last roughly 30 minutes to 1 hour. The frequency of visits and the length of treatment is determined by the team of providers who prescribe the treatment. The results are typically a result of the patient's commitment. When the patient follows the plan, does their exercises as often as suggested, and using the proper techniques, the treatment is typically very successful.

Before your appointment

It is a good idea to arrive at your physiotherapy appointment properly dressed. It is best that you wear snug comfortable clothing that doesn't restrict your movement. It is also a good idea to bring your insurance card, a form of identification, the prescription that your physician gave you, and if needed, your co-pay.

Faq's about physiotherapy and rehab

Do I need to see a physician before I can receive physiotherapy?

Yes. All Physiotherapy patients have been prescribed treatment from their physician prior to their therapy being scheduled.

What is the difference between chiropractors and physiotherapists?

Our providers perform a comprehensive analysis of a range of motion, including identifying the joints involved, tissue limitations, muscular imbalances, and structural pathologies. A chiropractor will treat the spine and are able to order special tests like X-rays, MRIs, and blood tests.

Chapter 9

Sciatica

Struggling with sciatica?

One of the most common appearances in the ER is someone suffering from sciatica. Unfortunately, millions of people experience pain from sciatica and don't know how to relieve it. Without treatment, your sciatica problem will continue to worsen.

How do you know you have sciatica? Most of our patients say they experience mild to severe pain running up and down the legs and feet. They will say that the pain comes at random times, and it also worsens as time goes on.

Sciatica

The main parts of your spine that usually causes sciatica is the pelvic and lumbar areas. With help from our team, we can pinpoint the location of the issue. Once we have done this, the next task is fixing the underlying issue with the manipulation of the spine and discs, specific stretches and exercises and possible injections from our Nurse Practitioner to accelerate healing.

Many tasks, as simple as bending over to pick up something, have resulted in intense pain for sciatica suffering patients. This sciatica attack can be worrisome, but the reality is that sciatica can develop for years. This is also the case with other spine issues.

Sciatica treatment and time frame

Depending on the severity and location of the condition, sciatica can be a quick to the long-term recovery process. A common correlation is that the longer the condition had to develop, the longer it will take to correct the issue. However, because of our Doctor's extensive schooling and experience they can clear up the issue in a quicker time than it took to develop.

With a low rate of success and high amounts of tries, you would think back surgery should be avoided. You deserve better results. Back surgery has shown that only 15 percent of people are positively affected by back surgery in a 5-year time period.

At Ridgeview Medical, we are here to naturally fix your sciatica. Don't hesitate to give us a call today if you're looking for the relief you deserve!

Chapter 10

Trigger Point Injections

Trigger Point Injections

Trigger point injection is a procedure used to treat the areas of muscle that are in pain and contain trigger points or knots of muscle that are created when muscles cannot relax. It is possible to feel these knots under the skin. It is fairly common that trigger points irritate the nerves around them and cause a pain that is felt in another part of the body, known as a referred pain. Our team has found some patient complaints respond very well to this form of treatment.

Understanding trigger point injections

The trigger point injection procedure consists of injecting a solution through a small needle into the patient's trigger point problem area. The solution contains a local anesthetic such as Lidocaine. When injected, the trigger point is made inactive, and the pain is alleviated. Usually, a brief course of treatment will result in sustained relief. Injections are given in a doctor's office and usually take just a few minutes. Several sites may be injected in one visit.

Trigger point injection treatment

Trigger point injections are used to treat many muscle groups, especially those in the arms, legs, lower back, and neck. In addition, trigger point injection can be used to treat fibromyalgia and tension headaches. Trigger point injection is also used to alleviate myofascial pain syndrome (chronic pain involving tissue that surrounds muscle) that does not respond to other treatments. However, the effectiveness of trigger point injections for treating myofascial pain is still under study.

Chapter 11

What Patients Are Saying

Pam W.

Dr. Martin is a wonderful knowledgeable healer. When I first started coming to him I was in extreme pain and found moving, walking, sleeping very difficult. I had relief after the first session, and now My overall health has greatly improved, I am no longer in pain. Dr. Martin has taught me so much about the body and healing, the quality of my life has greatly improved! I did not have to go on painkillers or have surgery. I give Dr Martin 5 stars out of 5!

Ryan H.

My family has been seeing Dr. Martin for years. He has helped me and my wife through grade 2-3 pinched nerves and we've continued on maintenance plans to keep healthy and are happy to report no relapses. The office is clean and inviting and Kasey is great with scheduling and a welcoming smile every visit.

Michelle M.

After years in pain, I finally have hope. Dr. Martin is both patient and thorough, Kasey at the front desk is super helpful. I highly recommend.

Patrick B.

Dr. Holcomb and Dr. Martin are true compassionate and caring professionals. I always feel very confident with their advice for my health. The office is very pleasant and clean. I highly recommend their care.

Azita C.

I had a great experience at Ridgeview Medical in Plano. The Doctors there really care! My back pain is so much better. This is the place to come for regenerative medicine like stem cell, PRP and rehabilitation! It works.

Tracey W.

Dr. Martin explained to me exactly what is going on with my spine. He showed me why the exercises I am doing are helping to repair and reverse damage incurred over a lifetime. I already have more mobility in my neck. So happy this can be repaired and not covered up with pain killers!

Amazing team - extremely kind and supportive. Thank you Dr. Martin AND Kasey!

William G.

Ever since starting treatment I have noticed dramatic changes in mobility, energy, and quality of sleep. I've also noticed that the chronic aches and pains from a back injury have completely subsided. I appreciate how Dr Martin and staff are extremely thorough in explaining the entire process of your treatment plan. I wish I would have started a lot sooner.

Hyungsup C.

Dr. Martin is great and helped me get rid of my chronic shoulder pain. Kasey is just as awesome as she does an amazing job shuffling my appoints around through my ever changing work schedule. Absolutely give them a call if you have any back or neck issues.

Troy K.

Dr. Martin & Casey take care of you with new and innovative ways to get your mobility back. When I started this a couple of months ago I didn't expect the return I got looking back on it today. I am totally invest in taking care of my body and Dr. Martin is very insightful on how to keep you moving. Check them out today I can promise you wont be disappointed.

William J.

Friendly staff and relatable doctor who is willing to go over every detail of your treatment plan with you. No detail is spared!

Sarah M.

Dr. Martin and Kacey are both phenomenal. Kaycee is so friendly every time I walk in the door and Dr. Martin has really helped improve my back and neck. I used to have headaches daily and now they are completely gone. My whole body feels better. They are really about improving your health as a whole and helping your entire wellbeing.

Deborah J.

I love all my visits to Dr. Martin's office. He is the most kind and gentle man. He really cares about your needs and problems. I also love his seminars. They're very professional and educational - mind opening

Whitney S.

I've struggled with spinal and neck problems for years and wasn't getting any relief. I was advised by a friend to try this place out and I'm glad I listened! Dr. Martin goes really deep in depth in explaining your issues/problems. You don't have to go elsewhere for your X-rays because he takes them right at the office and goes over it with you. He's truly passionate about healing his patients and goes and beyond to make sure that you are comfortable. I'm already two weeks in and this is the first time in the past few years that I've been able to rest well at night. Give him a shot I promise you won't regret it?

Lisa G.

I highly recommend Dr Martin and his staff they are a close family orientated practice. Since I have been going a lot of my issues are starting to get resolved. Very informative with one-on-one care. Worth the time and money to come see them. Family friendly with a knowledgeable office and staff. Thank you for taking such great care of me.

Alexander P.

Dr. Jarrad is fantastic. He eliminated most of my aches and pains and increased my flexibility in just a few short sessions. He uses a gentle touch technique to address each area and really improved my quality of life. I feel 15 years younger!

Don't wait like I did. I think back on all the things I missed out on because I did not want to aggravate my back or shoulders. There is no getting those days back. Fortunately, now I can take advantage of all the days ahead.

Thank you Dr. Jarrad!

April C.

He's a wonderful doctor that has help me through my chronic pain. I recommend anyone and everyone to come see him

Keala G.

Best overall experience! Everyone treats you like family and they TRUELY care about your recovery!

Robert O.

Dr. Martin is a kindhearted young man with a passion for helping folks, and his support staff is awesome! I spent thousands trying to deal with agonizing pelvic pain...MRI's, CT's, injections, urology drugs, neurology drugs, nothing worked. Then I go see Dr. Martin and I'm improving each week. What a blessing! Don't wait, go see him!

Sandra C.

I could barely turn my neck and had horrible lower back pain with pain radiating down my leg. Dr. Martin has helped me tremendously with my back and neck issues. I can't thank him enough! His staff is very friendly and helpful.

Chapter 12

Supportive Studies

UMBILICAL CORD / WHARTON'S JELLY

Immunosuppressive properties of mesenchymal stromal cells derived from amnion, placenta, Wharton's jelly and umbilical cord.

https://www.ncbi.nlm.nih.gov/pubmed/23176558

- CONCLUSION:
- The results obtained from this study suggest that MSC from amnion, placenta, Wharton's jelly and umbilical cord can therefore be potentially used for substituting BM-MSC in several therapeutic applications, including the treatment of GvHD.

Immune characterization of mesenchymal stem cells in human umbilical cord Wharton's jelly and derived cartilage cells

https://www.sciencedirect.com/science/article/abs/pii/S0008874912001220

- The hWJMSC has very low immunogenicity and good potential to tolerate rejection. Their intermediate state between adult and embryonic stem cells makes them an ideal candidate for reprogramming to the pluripotent status.

A comparison of human bone marrow-derived mesenchymal stem cells and human umbilical cord-derived mesenchymal stromal cells for cartilage tissue engineering.

https://www.ncbi.nlm.nih.gov/pubmed/19260778

- Therefore, it was concluded that hUCMSCs may be a desirable option for use as a mesenchymal cell source for fibrocartilage tissue engineering, based on abundant type I collagen and aggrecan production of hUCMSCs in a 3D matrix, although further investigation of signals that best promote type II collagen production of hUCMSCs is warranted for hyaline cartilage engineering.

Comparison of human mesenchymal stem cells derived from dental pulp, bone marrow, adipose tissue, and umbilical cord tissue by gene expression.

https://www.ncbi.nlm.nih.gov/pubmed/24145770

- Comparison of human mesenchymal stem cells derived from dental pulp, bone marrow, adipose tissue, and umbilical cord tissue by gene expression.
- All MSCs tested were phenotypically similar and of fibroblastoid morphology. DP-MSCs and UBC-MSCs were more proliferative than bone marrow BM-MSCs and AT-MSCs.

Ultrastructural and immunocytochemical analysis of multilineage differentiated human dental pulp- and umbilical cord-derived mesenchymal stem cells.

https://www.ncbi.nlm.nih.gov/pubmed/21124001

- Our results demonstrate, at the biochemical and ultrastructural level, that DPSC display at least bilineage potential, whereas UCSC, which are developmentally more primitive cells, show trilineage potential. We emphasize that transmission electron microscopical analysis is useful to elucidate detailed structural information and provides indisputable evidence of differentiation. These findings highlight their potential therapeutic value for cell-based tissue engineering.

Endothelial differentiation of Wharton's jelly-derived mesenchymal stem cells in comparison with bone marrow-derived mesenchymal stem cells.

https://www.ncbi.nlm.nih.gov/pubmed/19375653

- CONCLUSION: These results showed that UC-MSCs had higher endothelial differentiation potential than BM-MSCs. Therefore, UC-MSCs are more favorable choice than BM-MSCs for neovascularization of engineered tissues.

Feasibility, Safety, and Tolerance of Mesenchymal Stem Cell Therapy for Obstructive Chronic Lung Allograft Dysfunction

https://stemcellsjournals.onlinelibrary.wiley.com/doi/10.1002/sctm.17-0198

- Conclusion: The results of our study suggest it is safe and feasible to provide cell therapy with intravenous infusion of bone marrow-derived MSCs to lung transplant recipients with moderate obstructive CLAD, warranting future studies to assess the effectiveness of this therapy for management of acute or chronic graft dysfunction.

Human umbilical cord mesenchymal stem cells: a new era for stem cell therapy.

https://www.ncbi.nlm.nih.gov/pubmed/25622293

- The human umbilical cord is a promising source of mesenchymal stem cells (HUCMSCs). Unlike bone marrow stem cells, HUCMSCs have a painless collection procedure and faster self-renewal properties. Different derivation protocols may provide different amounts and populations of stem cells. Stem cell populations have also been reported in other compartments of the umbilical cord, such as the cord lining, perivascular tissue, and Wharton's jelly. HUCMSCs are noncontroversial sources compared to embryonic stem cells. They can differentiate into the three germ layers that promote tissue repair and modulate immune responses and anticancer properties. Thus, they are attractive autologous or allogenic agents for the treatment of malignant and nonmalignant solid and soft cancers. HUCMCs also can be the feeder layer for embryonic stem cells or other pluripotent stem cells.

Comparative Characterization of Cells from the Various Compartments of the Human Umbilical Cord Shows that the Wharton's Jelly Compartment Provides the Best Source of Clinically Utilizable Mesenchymal Stem Cells

https://neomatrixmedical.com/wp-content/uploads/2018/05/2015-Singapore-Mesenchymal-Stem-Cells-From-Umbilical-Cord-Tissue-Are-Best-in-Clinical-Applicatoins-2.pdf

• Taken together, it appears that MSCs from the WJ are more superior than those from the PV, SA, AM and MC in terms of clinical utility and research value because (i) their isolation is simple, quick and easy to standardize, (i) they have lesser non-stem cell contaminants (iii) they are rich in stemness characteristics, (iv) they can be generated in large numbers with minimal manipulation, (v) they are proliferative and (vi) have broad and efficient differentiation potential.

They will thus be stable and attractive candidates for research and future cell-based therapies when derived, propagated and characterized correctly. Our results show that when isolating MSCs from the UC, the WJ should be the preferred compartment, and a standardized method of derivation must be used so as to make meaningful comparisons of data between research groups.

Different populations and sources of human mesenchymal stem cells (MSC): A comparison of adult and neonatal tissue-derived MSC

https://neomatrixmedical.com/wp-content/uploads/2018/05/Comparison-of-Adult-and-Neonatal-Tissue-MSCs_Hass_2011-copy.pdf

- In contrast, the umbilical cord tissue or Wharton's jelly is an excellent source for isolating MSC [103-105]. Source-related features of MSC might directly contribute to the diversity of opinions regarding the mechanisms (soluble factors versus cell-to-cell contact) of MSC-mediated immunomodulation

The umbilical cord matrix is a better source of mesenchymal stem cells (MSC) than the umbilical cord blood

https://neomatrixmedical.com/wp-content/uploads/2018/05/Umbilical-Cord-vs-Blood-MSC-source.Zeddou2010-copy.pdf

- Conclusion According to the critical parameters of sample selection described in the literature, and using different culture media proposed to enhance the growth of MSC, in parallel with the use of different methods of cell isolation, we were not able to establish MSC cultures from more than one out of 15 UCB samples. Given the high frequency of MSC in UCM, we hypothesize that there may be MSC contamination while collecting cord blood. This may explain the rare described cases where MSC isolation from UCB has been possible. However, it could not be ascertained whether the collection method may have caused the disappearance of circulating MSC from the cord blood MNC compartment in favor of the endothelial/subendothelial layer of the UCM. Anyway, UCB can be excluded as a reliable source of MSC in favor of the richer and more reproducible source that is the UCM.

Umbilical Cord Tissue Offers the Greatest Number of Harvestable Mesenchymal Stem Cells for Research and Clinical Application: A Literature Review of Different Harvest Sites

https://neomatrixmedical.com/wp-content/uploads/2018/05/Umbilical-Cord-WJ-greatest-_-MSC.VANGSNESS2015-copy.pdf

- Large variations in cell harvest yields remain for each major tissue site for MSCs as reported in the literature to date. Reviewed research supports the understanding that placental tissue provides the highest concentration of cells whereas adipose tissue offers the highest levels of autologous cells. Consequently, considerations must be made regarding the non-autologous nature of umbilical cord derived stem cells, as well as the increased post-harvest processing required for adipose-derived stem cells, for the purposes of research and clinical application.

Discarded Wharton's Jelly of the Human Umbilical Cord: A Viable Source for Mesenchymal Stem Cells

https://neomatrixmedical.com/wp-content/uploads/2018/05/Umbilical-Cord-WJ-viable-MSC.Watson2015-copy.pdf

- In particular, WJ is a predominantly good source of cells because MSCs in WJ (WJ-MSC) are maintained in a very early embryological phase and therefore have retained some of the primitive stemness properties. WJ-MSCs can easily differentiate into a plethora of cell types leading to a variety of applications. WJ-MCSs are still the ideal future for cell therapy; their properties of high proliferation capability and versatility to differentiate between three lineages allow them to lower immunogenicity and have the potential to treat an array of diseases and disorders

Umbilical Cord as Prospective Source for Mesenchymal Stem Cell-Based Therapy

https://neomatrixmedical.com/wp-content/uploads/2018/05/Umbilical-Cord-as-Prospective-Source-for-Mesenchymal-Stem-Cell-Based-Therapy-1.pdf

- Conclusion The human umbilical cord is a source of MSCs that have Currently isolated and cultured umbilical cord MSCs are a promising storage object of the leading biobanks of the world, and the number of registered clinical trials on their use is currently growing.

Human Umbilical Cord-Derived Mesenchymal Stem Cells Do Not Undergo Malignant Transformation during Long-Term Culturing in Serum-Free Medium

https://neomatrixmedical.com/wp-content/uploads/2018/05/Human-Umbilical-Cord-Derived-Mesenchymal-Stem-Cells-Do-Not-Undergo-Malignant-Tr.pdf

- Results Flow cytometry analysis showed that very high expression was detected for CD105, CD73, and CD90 and very low expression for CD45, CD34, CD14, CD79a, and HLA-DR. MSCs could differentiate into osteocytes, chondrocytes, and adipocytes in vitro. There was no obvious chromosome elimination, displacement, or chromosomal imbalance as determined from the guidelines of the International System for Human Cytogenetic Nomenclature. Telomerase activity was down-regulated significantly when the culture time was prolonged. Further, no tumors formed in rats injected with hUC-MSCs (P) cultured in serum-free and in serum containing conditions. Conclusion Our data showed that hUC-MSCs met the International Society for Cellular Therapy sandards for conditions of long-term in vitro culturing at P . Since hUC-MSCs can be safely expanded in vitro and are not susceptible to malignant transformation in serum-free medium, these cells are suitable for cell therapy.

Comparative Analysis Of Bone Marrow and Wharton's Jelly Mesenchymal Stem/Stromal Cells

http://www.bloodjournal.org/content/122/21/1212?sso-checked=true

- Taken together WJ-MSCs display decreased cellular senescence after extended in vitro culture, increased proliferative capacity and reduced potential to differentiate in vitro to adipocytes and osteocytes, as compared to BM-MSCs. The last two observations can be explained, at least partly, by the aberrant expression of Wnt-signaling molecules in WJ-MSCs. The emerging role of Wnt-signaling pathway in WJ-MSC biology is currently under investigation.

Mesenchymal stem cells derived from Wharton's Jelly of the umbilical cord: biological properties and emerging clinical applications.

https://www.ncbi.nlm.nih.gov/pubmed/23279098

- Thus, there is accumulating interest in identifying alternative sources for MSCs. To this end MSCs obtained from the Wharton's Jelly (WJ) of umbilical cords (UC) have gained much attention over the last years since they can be easily isolated, without any ethical concerns, from a tissue which is discarded after birth. Furthermore WJ-derived MSCs represent a more primitive population than their adult counterparts, opening new perspectives for cell-based therapies. In this review we will at first give an overview of the biology of WJ-derived UC-MSCs. Then their potential application for the treatment of cancer and immune mediated disorders, such graft versus host disease (GVHD) and systemic lupus erythematosus (SLE) will be discussed, and finally their putative role as feeder layer for ex vivo hematopoietic stem cell (HSC) expansion will be pointed out.

Wharton's Jelly Derived Mesenchymal Stem Cells: Future of Regenerative Medicine? Recent Findings and Clinical Significance

https://www.hindawi.com/journals/bmri/2015/430847/

- Taken together, the clinical implication of oxidative stress, telomere length, DNA damage and disease is impaired therapeutic potential of MSC isolated from aged patients. These changes in MSC biology indicate that aged patients may require an alternative source of stem cells for treatment. The high efficiency of WJ-MSC recovery, the minimal ethical concerns associated with its acquirement and use, low immunogenicity, and the fact that they are from healthy, young donors make them an ideal source of MSC for autologous and allogeneic applications.

Wharton's jelly as a reservoir of peptide growth factors.
https://www.ncbi.nlm.nih.gov/pubmed/16226124

- The amounts of peptide growth factors calculated per microgram of DNA are distinctly higher in Wharton's jelly in comparison to the umbilical cord artery. Western blot analysis demonstrated that almost the entire amount of these factors is bound to high molecular weight components. Since the number of cells in Wharton's jelly is very low and the amounts of extracellular matrix components are very high, it is concluded that the cells are strongly stimulated by peptide growth factors to produce large amounts of collagen and glycosaminoglycans.

NEUROPATHY

Enhanced neuro-therapeutic potential of Wharton's Jelly-derived mesenchymal stem cells in comparison with bone marrow mesenchymal stem cells culture.
https://www.ncbi.nlm.nih.gov/pubmed/26971678

- In order to determine the variable responses to MSCs therapy, the present study examines and compares the adhesive stromal cells from immature perinatal tissues—umbilical cord Wharton's Jelly (WJ-MSC) and from adult, healthy donors of bone marrow origin (BM-MSC).

- WJ-MSC represent an example of immature type of "pre-MSC" population with exceptionally high commitment to neural differentiation.
- WJ-MSC exhibit a higher proliferation rate, a greater expansion capability and enhanced neurotrophic factors expression in comparison to BM-MSC.
- Hypoxia conditions accelerated WJ cells growth together with a regression of cell differentiation/maturation.
- The cultures of hypo-oxygenated BM-MSC do not express any of the phenomena mentioned above, except for the moderate stimulation of cell growth.

Human umbilical cord Wharton's Jelly-derived mesenchymal stem cells differentiation into nerve-like cells.
https://www.ncbi.nlm.nih.gov/pubmed/16336835

- CONCLUSIONS:MSCs could be isolated from human umbilical cord Wharton's Jelly. They were capable of differentiating into nerve-like cells using Salvia miltiorrhiza or beta-mercaptoethanol. The induced MSCs not only underwent morphologic changes, but also expressed the neuron-related genes and neuronal cell markers. They may represent an alternative source of stem cells for central nervous system cell transplantation

Perspectives of employing mesenchymal stem cells from the Wharton's jelly of the umbilical cord for peripheral nerve repair.

https://www.ncbi.nlm.nih.gov/pubmed/24083432

• Mesenchymal stem cells (MSCs) from Wharton's jelly present high plasticity and low immunogenicity, turning them into a desirable form of cell therapy for the injured nervous system. Their isolation, expansion, and characterization have been performed from cryopreserved umbilical cord tissue. The MSCs from Wharton's jelly delivered through tested biomaterials should be regarded a potentially valuable tool to improve clinical outcome especially after trauma to sensory nerves. In addition, these cells represent a noncontroversial source of primitive mesenchymal progenitor cells, which can be harvested after birth, cryogenically stored, thawed, and expanded for therapeutic uses.

Stem Cell Technology for Neurodegenerative Diseases

https://www.ncbi.nlm.nih.gov/pmc/articles/PMC3177143/

• Cellular therapies offer great promise for the treatment of these diseases, and research progress to date supports the utilization of stem cells to offer cellular replacement and/or provide environmental enrichment to attenuate neurodegeneration. In diseases where specific subpopulations of cells or widespread neuronal loss are present, cellular replacement may reproduce or stabilize neuronal networks. In addition, environmental enrichment may provide neurotrophic support to remaining cells or prevent the production or accumulation of toxic factors that harm neurons. In many cases, cellular therapies provide beneficial effects through both mechanisms.

Human mesenchymal stem cells improve the neurodegeneration of femoral nerve in a diabetic foot ulceration rats

https://www.sciencedirect.com/science/article/abs/pii/S0304394015003377?via%3Dihub

• These data suggested that hMSCs-UC-treatment partially reverse the neuronal degeneration and nerve function of FN, which might be contributed by the upregulation of NGF with dramatic angiogenesis in FN-innervated gastrocnemius, consequently reversing neuronal structure and function, preventing or curing foot ulceration.

Stem Cells for the Treatment of Neuropathic Pain

http://www.japmnet.com/uploadfile/2017/0121/20170121044012254.full.pdf

- Stem cell transplantation can effectively relieve neuropathic pain under different pathological conditions. However, it is interesting to point out that peripheral neuropathic pain seems to be more responsive to stem cell therapy than SCI (Spinal Cord Injury) induced chronic pain. Moreover, stem cell treatment does not always exert positive results in SCI- induced chronic pain (e.g. aggravating pain above the lesion spinal cord segment).

Mesenchymal stem cells to treat diabetic neuropathy: a long and strenuous way from bench to the clinic

https://www.researchgate.net/publication/306435063_Mesenchymal_stem_cells_to_treat_diabetic_neuropathy_a_long_and_strenuous_way_from_bench_to_the_clinic

- CONCLUSION DN (Diabetic Neuropathy) frequently leads to foot ulcers and ultimately limb amputations without effective clinical therapy. DN is characterized by reduced vascularity in the peripheral nerves and deficiency in angiogenic and neurotrophic factors. Only delivering neurotrophic or angio-genic factors for treatment in the form of protein or gene therapy is very modest if not ineffective. MSCs have been highlighted as a new emerging regenerative therapy owing to their multipotency for DN.MSCs reverse manifestations of DN, repair tissue, and anti-hyperglycemia. MSCs also paracrinely secrete neurotrophic factors, angio-genic factors, cytokines, and immunomodulatory substances to ameliorate DN.

Mesenchymal Stem Cells as a Prospective Therapy for the Diabetic Foot

https://www.ncbi.nlm.nih.gov/pmc/articles/PMC5102750/

- In summary, MSC transplantation is a new technology that can be used to treat the diabetic foot and is a well-studied topic in the field of angiogenesis. MSCs have high proliferative and self-renewal capabilities in addition to the ability to differentiate into multiple types of cells, including VECs, SMCs, and astrocytes and, to a lesser extent, oligodendrocytes and Schwann cells, after transplantation. The transplanted stem cells regulate the immune system by influencing the immune responses of T cells, natural killer cells, macrophages, and dendritic cells, and they participate in diabetic wound healing. Via both endocrine and paracrine effects and the secretion of angiogenic factors, cytokines and neurotrophic factors that promote angiogenesis, the blood flow in the local tissue recovers, and neurological lesions are healed. MEX also participate in the wound healing process via the effects of the mRNA, miRNA, and protein molecules which they contain (Figures (Figures1,1, ,2,2, and and3).3). Although certain researchers argue that transplanted MSCs can also recover islet β cell dysfunction and maintain balanced blood glucose levels, these phenomena seem to lack supporting evidence [172]. In animals with diabetic feet and in clinical trials, the transplantation of MSCs has led to positive results, and, in short-term follow-ups, there have been no significant adverse reactions or serious complications. The MSC transplantation technique has therefore been successfully developed, and it provides a basis for clinical applications involving stem cell transplantation to treat the diabetic foot.

Effect of subcutaneous treatment with human umbilical cord blood-derived multipotent stem cells on peripheral neuropathic pain in rats

https://www.ncbi.nlm.nih.gov/pmc/articles/PMC5343048/

- We demonstrated that hUCB-MSCs showed a significant improvement in animal models for neuropathic pain after intraplantar, subcutaneous transplantation. It seems that hUCB-MSCs transplantation cause secretion of

TIMP-2, which inhibits MMP 2 activation that otherwise produces neuropathic pain symptoms, via IL-βcleavage and activation of p-ERK in astrocytes [21]. This finding was indirectly confirmed by expression of c-fos and CGRP, which are generally used as stress markers p-ERK, which is upstream of c-fos and CGRP. Among three animal models for neuropathic pain, spinal cord cells positive for c-fos, CGRP, p-ERK, p-p 38, MMP-9 and MMP 2 were significantly decreased in only CCI model of hUCB-MSCs-grafted rats. The CCI model has been extensively used for many neuropathic studies because it closely mimics the clinical nerve injury conditions and pain nature such as complex regional pain syndrome type 2

Perspectives of employing mesenchymal stem cells from the Wharton's jelly of the umbilical cord for peripheral nerve repair.

https://www.ncbi.nlm.nih.gov/pubmed/24083432

• Mesenchymal stem cells (MSCs) from Wharton's jelly present high plasticity and low immunogenicity, turning them into a desirable form of cell therapy for the injured nervous system. Their isolation, expansion, and characterization have been performed from cryopreserved umbilical cord tissue.

ORTHOPEDIC CONDITIONS / SPORTS INJURIES

Characteristics of mesenchymal stem cells derived from Wharton's jelly of human umbilical cord and for fabrication of non-scaffold tissue-engineered cartilage.
https://www.ncbi.nlm.nih.gov/pubmed/23899897

- The human WMSCs express characteristics of pre-chondrocytes, low immunogenicity and are easy to be obtained with higher purity because there have no hematopoietic cells in Wharton's jelly, so it may be a new seed cells more suitable for constructing tissue-engineered cartilage.

Mesenchymal stem cells in regenerative medicine: Focus on articular cartilage and intervertebral disc regeneration
https://www.sciencedirect.com/science/article/pii/S1046 2315300918?via%3Dihub

- In addition, WJSCs has several advantages that make them an attractive choice for use in tissue engineering and regenerative medicine. WJSCs (i) are a relatively young cell type compared to most other MSCs, (ii) have no ethical concerns unlike ESCs, (iii) can be harvested painlessly unlike bone-marrow MSCs, (iv) share few embryonic features, (v) have high cell proliferation, (vi) have wide differentiation potential, (vii) are hypo-immunogenic and (viii) are non-tumorigenic [61], [62], [63], [64], [65], [66], [67]. Developmentally, the umbilical cord and its contents are embryonic in nature as it arises from the epiblast, which also give rise to the three primordial germ layers, the amnion and the allantois. Therefore, WJSCs come to occupy an intermediate position between the most versatile pluripotent ESCs/iPSCs and adult tissue specific MSCs, which might explain the presence of some embryonic stem features and increased stemness.

• WJSCs, by their inherent nature have high hyaluronic acid, sulfated glycosaminoglycans (GAGs) and collagen expression [73], which to some extent reflect native cartilage tissue. Moreover, uses of WJSCs following their differentiation into multiple cell types as reported by many different research groups, with some progressing on to clinical trials is encouraging [74], [75], [76] and justify the use of WJSCs in cartilage regeneration procedures.

Regeneration of Full-Thickness Rotator Cuff Tendon Tear After Ultrasound-Guided Injection With Umbilical Cord Blood-Derived Mesenchymal Stem Cells in a Rabbit Model

https://stemcellsjournals.onlinelibrary.wiley.com/doi/10.5966/sctm.2015-0040

• Conclusion UCB-derived MSC injection under ultrasound guidance without surgical repair or bioscaffold resulted in the partial healing of full-thickness rotator cuff tendon tears in a rabbit model. Histology revealed that UCB-derived MSCs induced regeneration of rotator cuff tendon tears and that the regenerated tissue was predominantly composed of type I collagens. In addition, motion analysis showed better walking capacity after MSC injection than HA or normal saline injection. These results suggest that ultrasound-guided UCB-derived MSC injection may be a useful conservative treatment for full-thickness rotator cuff tendon tear repair.

Human umbilical cord-derived mesenchymal stem cells reduce monosodium iodoacetate-induced apoptosis in cartilage

https://www.ncbi.nlm.nih.gov/pmc/articles/PMC5968746/

- Based on the present findings, we conclude that HUCMSCs can fulfill MSC characteristics with mesoderm differentiation capability. HUCMSCs can assist MIA-treated mice in regeneration of hyaline cartilage and/or repair of cartilage damage and in ameliorating cartilage apoptosis. These effects can be associated with motor behavioral improvement. Thus, HUCMSCs may be a feasible source for stem cell treatment for OA cartilage repair.

Effects of insulin-like growth factor-induced Wharton jelly mesenchymal stem cells toward chondrogenesis in an osteoarthritis model.

https://www.ncbi.nlm.nih.gov/pubmed/30140415

- Effects of insulin-like growth factor-induced Wharton jelly mesenchymal stem cells toward chondrogenesis in an osteoarthritis model.

CONCLUSION: The IGF1-induced WJMSCs were capable to enhance chondrogenesis, indicated by increased expression of SOX9 and COL2 and decreased expression of ADAMTS1, ADAMTS5, MMP3, MMP1, and RANKL. These findings can be further used in the osteoarthritis treatment.

Effect of nicotine on the proliferation and chondrogenic differentiation of the human Wharton's jelly mesenchymal stem cells.

https://www.ncbi.nlm.nih.gov/pubmed/28372298

• Effect of nicotine on the proliferation and chondrogenic differentiation of the human Wharton's jelly mesenchymal stem cells. CONCLUSIONS: At the concentration used, nicotine had an adverse effect on the proliferation and chondrogenic differentiation of hWJ-MSCs which was probably impaired through a α7 nAChR mediation

Human Wharton's Jelly Mesenchymal Stem Cells Maintain the Expression of Key Immunomodulatory Molecules When Subjected to Osteogenic, Adipogenic and Chondrogenic Differentiation In Vitro: New Perspectives for Cellular Therapy

https://neomatrixmedical.com/wp-content/uploads/2018/12/Human-whartons-jelly-MSCs-maintain-the-expression-of-key-immunomodulatory.pdf

• Human Wharton's Jelly Mesenchymal Stem Cells Maintain the Expression of Key Immunomodulatory Molecules When Subjected to Osteogenic, Adipogenic and Chondrogenic Differentiation In Vitro: New Perspectives for Cellular Therapy "This strongly suggests that also after the acquisition of a mature phenotype, WJ-MSCs-derived cells may maintain their immune privilege. This evidence, which deserves much work to be confirmed in vivo and in other MSCs populations, may provide a formal proof of the good results globally achieved with WJMSCs as cellular therapy vehicle."

Cartilage Repair in the Knee Using Umbilical Cord Wharton's Jelly–Derived Mesenchymal Stem Cells Embedded Onto Collagen Scaffolding and Implanted Under Dry Arthroscopy

https://www.ncbi.nlm.nih.gov/pmc/articles/PMC5852271/

- Cartilage Repair in the Knee Using Umbilical Cord Wharton's Jelly–Derived Mesenchymal Stem Cells Embedded Onto Collagen Scaffolding and Implanted Under Dry Arthroscop

- Although WJ-MSCs are allogeneically sourced, they are considered weakly immunogenic or non-immunogenic because of the low expression of HLA class I. The ability of these cells to promote chondrogenesis, without eliciting an immunogenic response, makes them an excellent candidate for providing cell-based cartilage repair in an off-the-shelf fashion. Moreover, use of WJ-MSCs for cartilage repair in older patients will address concerns related to MSC number and immunomodulatory capacity with autologous harvest in aging patients, making this technique a promising advancement in the treatment of cartilage injury for this demographic

Role of mesenchymal stem cells in osteoarthritis treatment

https://www.sciencedirect.com/science/article/pii/S2214031X17300074

- Role of mesenchymal stem cells in osteoarthritis treatment
- Without an effective cure, OA remains a significant clinical burden on our elderly population. The advancement of regenerative medicine and innovative stem cell technology offers a unique opportunity to treat this disease. In this review, we examine OA and the likely resolution with MSCs. MSCs have been one of the highlights in stem cell research in recent years. Although the application of MSCs in joint repair is well established, it is particularly exciting about MSCs being used for OA treatment.

Mesenchymal stem cells for cartilage regeneration in osteoarthritis

https://www.wjgnet.com/2218-5836/full/v8/i9/674.htm

- In summary, these studies show that MSCs can be employed successfully to treat mild to moderate OA through various ways. They provide alternative treatment options and treatment can start early during progression of OA. The traditional major surgeries used to treat late stages are expensive and come with risks. The less invasive techniques outlined in this minireview have revealed good outcomes, but the field merits further investigation. Superior outcome was evident with greater quantity of MSCs injected. Allogenic cells from healthy young donors can also be utilized. These findings have further empowered researchers to investigate the potentials of MSCs for tissue engineering and a number of clinical trials are now underway. Most of the emphasis on minimally invasive therapeutic alternatives including intraarticular injections of MSCs, aim to cut out cost and risks of major surgeries. Additional investigations are warranted to validate the safety and efficiency of different application before a standardized treatment regimen can be established.

EYE CONDITIONS

A Promising Tool in Retina Regeneration: Current Perspectives and Challenges When Using Mesenchymal Progenitor Stem Cells in Veterinary and Human Ophthalmological Applications

https://www.ncbi.nlm.nih.gov/pmc/articles/PMC5602072/

- Stem cells have been investigated in opthalmological research as a forthcoming tool for retinal degeneration. Mesenchymal stem cells have exhibited many advantages because of their multilineage differentiation potential, the ease in their culturing and their immunomodulatory properties which are crucial in retinal regeneration research. Current exploration has determined new mechanisms of regeneration and MSC protective capabilities, on degeneration of different types of retinal cell ad retinal vessels. Mesenchymal stem cell-derived microvesicles (MVs) allow for developments in future research and clinical applications as a result of their availability as well as the growth factors, miRNA and mRNA they possess. Studies have shown that the application of MVs in regenerative medicine proves to be very dynamic, which is directing clinical research in opthamology towards this domain of study. In the grand scheme of scientific interest, it is expected that MVs may have higher output and potential in retinal regeneration than stem cell therapies have so far, therefore it is anticipated that this research field will be moving further into this direction.

Therapeutic Potential of Mesenchymal Stem Cell-Derived Exosomes in the Treatment of Eye Diseases.
https://www.ncbi.nlm.nih.gov/pubmed/29774506

- Mesenchymal stem cells (MSCs) were, due to their immunomodulatory and pro-angiogenic characteristics, extensively explored as new therapeutic agents in cell-based therapy of uveitis, glaucoma, retinal and ocular surface diseases.Since it was recently revealed that exosomes play an important role in biological functions of MSCs, herewith we summarized current knowledge about the morphology, structure, phenotype and functional characteristics of MSC-derived exosomes emphasizing their therapeutic potential in the treatment of eye diseases. .In conclusion, MSC-derived exosomes represent potentially new therapeutic agents in the therapy of degenerative and inflammatory ocular diseases.

E.D. (Erectyle Dysfunction)

BDNF-hypersecreting human umbilical cord blood mesenchymal stem cells promote erectile function in a rat model of cavernous nerve electrocautery injury.

https://www.ncbi.nlm.nih.gov/pubmed/26577999

- CONCLUSIONS: Intracavernous injection of BDNF-hypersecreting hUCB-MSCs can enhance the recovery of erectile function, promote the CNs regeneration and inhibit corpus cavernosum fibrosis after CNEI in a rat model.

Erectile dysfunction treated with intracavernous stem cells: A promising new therapy?

https://www.ncbi.nlm.nih.gov/pubmed/30300133

- The main cause involved in the pathophysiology of erectile dysfunction is vascular damage related to endothelial and neuronal injury. The interest in stem cell therapy is justified by their capability to differentiate into specific damaged tissues, including endothelium and nervous tissue, and induction of the host own cell proliferation.

Stem-cell therapy for erectile dysfunction.

https://www.ncbi.nlm.nih.gov/pubmed/26558088

- RESULTS: Fifty-four papers were identified and contributed, either as an original research report or review thereof, to this review. Several preclinical studies addressed SC-based therapies for the recovery of erectile function caused by a variety of both chronic and acute conditions. Overall, these studies showed beneficial effects of SC therapy, while evidence on the mechanisms of action of SC therapy varied between studies. One clinical trial investigated the short-term effects of SC therapy in diabetic patients with ED. Two more clinical trials are currently recruiting patients.
- CONCLUSIONS: The rapidly expanding and highly promising body of preclinical work on SC-based medicine providing a potential cure for ED, rather than merely symptom relief, is indicative of the increasing interest in regenerative options for sexual medicine over the past decade. Clinical trials are currently recruiting patients to test the preclinical results in men with ED.

Stem Cell Therapy for Erectile Dysfunction: Progress and Future Directions.

https://www.ncbi.nlm.nih.gov/pubmed/27784560

- RESULTS: Several preclinical studies have addressed stem cell-based therapies for the recovery of erectile function following cavernous nerve injury and in Peyronie's disease, diabetes, aging, and hyperlipidemia. Overall, these studies have shown beneficial effects of stem cell therapy, while evidence on the mechanisms of action of stem cell therapy still varies between studies.

• While many authors propose engraftment and differentiation of stem cells, a recent paradigm shift toward paracrine mechanisms of action is observed

Multipotent stromal cell therapy for cavernous nerve injury-induced erectile dysfunction.

https://www.ncbi.nlm.nih.gov/pubmed/22145667

• RESULTS: MSCs from both bone marrow and adipose tissue have shown beneficial effects in a variety of animal models for ED. While MSC application in chronic disease models such as diabetes, aging, and hyperlipidemia may result in cell engraftment and possibly MSC differentiation, this observation has not been made in the acute CNI rat model. In the latter setting, MSC effects seem to be established by cell recruitment toward the major pelvic ganglion and local paracrine interaction with the host neural tissue.

• CONCLUSIONS: While the type of model may influence the mechanisms of action of this MSC-based therapy, MSCs generally display efficacy in various animal models for ED.

Stem cell therapies in post-prostatectomy erectile dysfunction: a critical review.

https://www.ncbi.nlm.nih.gov/pubmed/28263125

- CONCLUSION: MSC therapy consistently improved erectile functions after CNI. There seems to be a consensus on the disease model used and outcome evaluation however further studies focusing on immunologic response to MSCs, their mechanism of action and in vivo fate are needed before their widespread use in clinic.

Advances in stem cell research for the treatment of male sexual dysfunctions.

https://www.ncbi.nlm.nih.gov/pubmed/26759972

- SUMMARY: Evidence from preclinical studies has established stem cells as a potential curative treatment for erectile dysfunction and early phase clinical trials are currently performed.

Stem Cells in Male Sexual Dysfunction: Are We Getting Somewhere?

https://www.ncbi.nlm.nih.gov/pubmed/28041853

- CONCLUSION: Stem cells have an established efficacy in preclinical studies and early clinical trials. Studies are currently being published demonstrating the safety of intrapenile injection of autologous bone marrow- and adipose tissue-derived stem cells.

MSC-derived exosomes ameliorate erectile dysfunction by alleviation of corpus cavernosum smooth muscle apoptosis in a rat model of cavernous nerve injury.
https://www.ncbi.nlm.nih.gov/pubmed/30257719

- CONCLUSIONS: Exosomes isolated from MSCs culture supernatants by ultracentrifugation could ameliorate CNI-induced ED in rats by inhibiting apoptosis in CCSMCs, with similar potency to that observed in the MSCs-treated group. Therefore, this cell-free therapy has great potential for application in the treatment of CNI-induced ED for replacing cell therapy. MSC-derived exosomes ameliorate erectile dysfunction in a rat model of cavernous nerve injury.

Additional Research:

The following are research articles with promising results for auto-immune conditions, cancer, COPD, and other. Please note that we are excited about the future of stem cell therapy but we DO NOT offer treatment at Neo Matrix Medical for these conditions.

Treatment of Psoriasis with Mesenchymal Stem Cells
https://www.amjmed.com/article/S0002-9343(15)01043-8/fulltext

- Unexpectedly, his skin lesions, as well as engraftment, recovered day by day. Six months later, the patient's lymphoma underwent complete remission and his psoriasis was significantly relieved (Figure A.2). The skin returned to normal within 12 months (Figure A.3). Now the patient has been monitored for nearly 5 years. His condition remains stable, with no recurrence of lymphoma or psoriasis.

Neural differentiation and potential use of stem cells from the human umbilical cord for central nervous system transplantation therapy.
https://www.ncbi.nlm.nih.gov/pubmed/18241062

- Recent findings also suggest that neurons derived from cord stroma mesenchymal cells could alleviate movement disorders in hemiparkinsonian animal models. We review here the neurogenic potential of umbilical cord stem cells and discuss possibilities of their exploitation as an alternative to human embryonic stem cells or neural stem cells for transplantation therapy of traumatic CNS injury and neurodegenerative diseases.

Discarded Wharton's Jelly of the Human Umbilical Cord: A Viable Source for Mesenchymal Stem Cells
https://www.ncbi.nlm.nih.gov/pmc/articles/PMC4274214/

- WJ-MCSs are still the ideal future for cell therapy; their properties of high proliferation capability and versatility to differentiate between three lineages allow them to lower immunogenicity and have the potential to treat an array of diseases and disorders

   ◦ Diabetes… Also additional research suggests that WJ-MSC may have the potential to benefit in the direct treatment of diabetes mellitus [38]. By using markers that indicate when certain genes are expressed, models have shown that WJ-MSCs have the capability to differentiate into all sorts of pancreatic cells including the insulin-producing β cells [39]. Using immunohistochemistry and ELISA assays, a significantly greater amount of insulin and

C-peptide protein was released from the differentiated cells than from the undifferentiated cells.

○ Liver disease...Transplantation of WJ-MSCs has also been tested in liver fibrosis. Using carbon tetrachloride (CCl4), rats were experimentally induced display liver fibrosis and 4 weeks later received WJ-MSCs injections [22]. After an additional 4 weeks, there was a remarkable decrease in the liver fibrosis in the rats treated with WJ-MSCs as compared to the rats that were not treated with the WJ-MSCs. Some WJ-MSCs exhibited phenotypes of the liver, and those WJ-MSCs that did not differentiate had the capability to secrete cytokines that have the potential to restore liver function [23]. These observations indicate a multi-pronged reparative mechanism of WJ-MSCs involving specific lineage differentiation and therapeutic molecules that are key pathways towards tissue repair.

Human Wharton's Jelly-Derived Stem Cells Display Immunomodulatory Properties and Transiently Improve Rat Experimental Autoimmune Encephalomyelitis.

https://www.ncbi.nlm.nih.gov/pubmed/25310756

• Collectively, we show that WJ-MSCs have trophic support properties and effectively modulate immune cell functioning both in vitro and in the EAE model, suggesting WJ-MSC may hold promise for MS therapy.

Role of Nonmuscle Myosin II in Migration of Wharton's Jelly-Derived Mesenchymal Stem Cells.

https://www.ncbi.nlm.nih.gov/pubmed/25923805

- Role of Nonmuscle Myosin II in Migration of Wharton's Jelly-Derived Mesenchymal Stem Cells.
- It is the promise of regeneration and therapeutic applications that has sparked an interest in mesenchymal stem cells (MSCs). Following infusion, MSCs migrate to sites of injury or inflammation by virtue of their homing property.

Lung mesenchymal stem cells-derived extracellular vesicles attenuate the inflammatory profile of Cystic Fibrosis epithelial cells.

https://www.ncbi.nlm.nih.gov/pubmed/30076968

- We conclude that the anti-inflammatory and anti-oxidant efficacy of EVs (extra cellular vesicles) derived from lung MSCs could be mediated by up-regulation of the PPARγ axis, whose down-stream effectors (NF-kB and HO-1) are well-known modulators of these pathways.

- EVs could be a novel strategy to control the hyper-inflamed condition in Cystic Fibrosis.

Interaction of Wharton's jelly derived fetal mesenchymal cells with tumor cells.

https://www.ncbi.nlm.nih.gov/pubmed/24804889

- Currently, pre-clinical and clinical studies have demonstrated the importance of stem cell based therapies for the treatment of human diseases. Fetal Mesenchymal Stem Cells (Fetal MSCs) are potential candidates that can be utilized for the treatment of different types of cancer. Recently, Wharton's jelly (umbilical cord matrix) was proved to be a rich source of MSCs and they can be isolated by non-invasive methods such as Ficoll density gradient and antibodies coupled magnetic beads without any ethical issues. Documentation based on various literatures emphasized that fetal MSCs isolated from fetal umbilical cord possess beneficial activity in cancer therapy than adult MSCs. Specific markers of fetal MSCs such as tumor tropism (exhibit tumor microenvironments which act similar to anti inflammation immune cells) and low immunogenicity conferred them as a promising tool in gene therapy based oncology research. Based on these facts, this review summarizes the potential interaction of fetal mesenchymal stem cells with tumor cells and their use in clinical protocols.

Autologous Cellular Therapy and its Effects on COPD: A Pilot Study

https://lunginstitute.com/white-papers/autologous-stem-cell-therapy-and-its-effects-on-copd/

COPD Improves with Stem Cell Therapy

https://copdnewstoday.com/2016/06/28/lung-institute-review-stem-cells-not-a-miracle-cure-for-copd-but-still-improving-lives/

Stem cell therapies for chronic obstructive pulmonary disease: current status of pre-clinical studies and clinical trials

https://www.ncbi.nlm.nih.gov/pmc/articles/PMC5864644/

- In summary, the approaches discussed for regenerative therapies have demonstrated positive effects in COPD animal models and have been safe in clinical trials. However, greater effort must be taken to develop approaches that will lead towards a curing solution to COPD patients.

ADDITIONAL RESEARCH

Stem cell therapy in chronic obstructive pulmonary disease. How far is it to the clinic?

https://www.ncbi.nlm.nih.gov/pubmed/30245915

• Previous studies suggest that cell-based therapies and novel bioengineering approaches may be potential therapeutic strategies for lung repair and remodeling. In this paper, we review the current evidence of stem cell therapy in COPD.

The clinical use of regenerative therapy in COPD.

https://www.ncbi.nlm.nih.gov/pubmed/25548520

• Animal and human studies have demonstrated that tissue-specific stem cells and bone marrow-derived cells contribute to lung tissue regeneration and protection, and thus administration of exogenous stem/progenitor cells or humoral factors responsible for the activation of endogenous stem/progenitor cells may be a potent next-generation therapy for chronic obstructive pulmonary disease.

Concise Review: Clinical Prospects for Treating Chronic Obstructive Pulmonary Disease with Regenerative Approaches

https://www.ncbi.nlm.nih.gov/pmc/articles/PMC3659729/

•   Cell therapies using various stem cells have been extensively evaluated. The lung is one of the easiest organs in which to instill exogenous cells because cells can be applied through both the airway and circulation. In addition, most of the intravenously instilled cells are trapped within the pulmonary circulation; therefore, the efficacy of cell delivery is naturally high.

•   Mesenchymal stem cells (MSCs) are the most extensively evaluated candidates for clinical cell-based therapy. Many clinical trials using MSCs have been registered and are ongoing. Autologous MSCs are easily isolated from the bone marrow and other tissues. MSCs are expected to reduce inflammation and promote the repair process. These beneficial effects are thought to be based on the ability of MSCs to modulate the immune system and their capacity to produce growth factors and cytokines [49], such as keratinocyte growth factor, HGF, and prostaglandin E2.

•   Because of these anti-inflammatory effects, a phase II clinical trial using MSCs has been performed in moderate and severe COPD patients [50]. The trial successfully demonstrated the safety of cell therapies using MSCs and some reduction in the inflammatory response in COPD patients but did not show any beneficial effects on lung function. Additional studies, especially in early-stage COPD patients, are needed.

Stem cell therapy: the great promise in lung disease.
https://www.ncbi.nlm.nih.gov/pubmed/19124369

• The use of adult stem cells to help with lung regeneration and repair could be a newer technology in clinical and regenerative medicine. In fact, different studies have shown that bone marrow progenitor cells contribute to repair and remodeling of lung in animal models of progressive pulmonary hypertension. Therefore, lung stem cell biology may provide novel approaches to therapy and could represent a great promise for the future of molecular medicine. In fact, several diseases can be slowed or even blocked by stem cell transplantation.

Current Status of Stem Cells and Regenerative Medicine in Lung Biology and Diseases
https://www.ncbi.nlm.nih.gov/pmc/articles/PMC4208500/

• Exciting progress in each of these areas provides further understanding of lung biology and repair after lung injury and further a sound scientific basis for therapeutic use of cell therapies and bioengineering approaches in treatment of lung diseases

Lung Regeneration: Endogenous and Exogenous Stem Cell Mediated Therapeutic Approaches

https://www.ncbi.nlm.nih.gov/pmc/articles/PMC4730369/

• Much study, so far, has been done to evaluate MSC-mediated cell therapy in various lung conditions, albeit mostly in animal models. In this case, it is important to note that the bulk of studies suggest the infused MSCs exhibits reparative/healing effects mostly through paracrine or immunomodulatory effects on recipient lung tissue, but not by engraftment Thus, it is imperative to view MSC therapy as cell-based immunomodulatory therapy rather than as attempts to regenerate or reconstitute lung tissues [6]. Nonetheless, much effort has been taken to date to understand the molecular mechanisms of lung development, disease dynamics and its regenerative process.

Endogenous and exogenous stem cells: a role in lung repair and use in airway tissue engineering and transplantation

https://www.ncbi.nlm.nih.gov/pmc/articles/PMC3004872/

• Human amniotic fluid SCs (hAFSCs) and umbilical blood cord (UBC)-derived SCs are new cell resources for lung regeneration. Human umbilical cord blood is a promising source for human MSCs Recent advances in airway tissue engineering provide a good opportunity for the treatment of a wide range of lung defects. In addition to the respiratory failure cases mentioned above, SC-based therapies show great potential for new clinical applications against acute respiratory distress syndrome [72], asthma [73], and bronchopulmonary dysplasia [74]. At present, the therapeutic potential of SCs is intensively assessed in rodent models of these diseases, with the possibility of proceeding to clinical trials

Adult stem cells for chronic lung diseases
https://onlinelibrary.wiley.com/doi/full/10.1111/resp.12112
• Conclusion: As a self-repair mechanism, living organisms have stem cells that are attracted to sites of injury. Chronic injury as well as ageing could exhaust and impair stem cell reparative capacity as well as diminish number of available stem cells. The mechanism(s) by which alterations in the homeostasis of stem cells pools are involved in the pathogenesis of chronic lung diseases is unknown. If stem cell exhaustion and ageing is the cause of morbid states, stem

cell-based therapies will be able to prevent and treat them. Restoration of stem cells has shown promising therapeutic benefits for certain lung pathologies. Particularly, the immunomodulatory capacity of B-MSC has been shown to be beneficial for lung diseases with exacerbated inflammatory responses. However, a generalized use of B-MSC in chronic lung diseases must be considered with caution, and careful studies are still required to establish safety and efficacy of such use.

Lung regeneration using amniotic fluid mesenchymal stem cells

https://www.tandfonline.com/doi/abs/10.1080/21691401.2017.1337023?journalCode=ianb20

- In this review, we give an update on the use of amniotic fluid mesenchymal stem cells (AFMSCs) as an optimal source for lungs scaffold re-cellularization, due to their limitless accessibility and possibility for proliferation and differentiation. Further studies will be required in tissue engineering (TE) and regenerative medicine (RM), especially shifting our focus towards AFMSCs as a cell source for this regeneration.

Stem cell therapy for lung diseases: From fundamental aspects to clinical applications.

htttps://www.ncbi.nlm.nih.gov/pubmed/30084809

• This review summarizes the recent advances in stem cell treatments and the research efforts conducted through the application of stem cell therapy for respiratory system diseases. In particular, researchers have used animal models to gather data about treating lung injury by stem cell transplantation. This review concentrated on the findings about route, timing and adjustment of cell transplantation dose, optimum stem cell type selection and potency marker of cells as therapeutic agents.

Adult stem cells in the treatment of autoimmune diseases

https://academic.oup.com/rheumatology/article/45/10/1187/2255946

• The past decade has seen the introduction of many agents, especially biologics, which have allowed a more successful control of AD manifestations. However, the elusive aim of tolerance induction has not yet been achieved. It could be that through harnessing the complex and multifaceted potential of cellular-based therapies, especially HSCT, a 'resetting' of auto-aggressive immune reactions while maintaining protective immunity will be possible. In addition, the anti-proliferative and immunomodulatory properties of MSCs combined with their immunological privilege and seemingly low toxicity may offer a new strategy for controlling and protecting vital organs from inflammatory, destructive autoimmune reactions.

Treatment of severe autoimmune disease by stem-cell transplantation

https://www.nature.com/articles/nature03728

•	Transplantation of haematopoietic stem cells — cells capable of self renewing and reconstituting all types of blood cell — can treat numerous lethal diseases, including leukaemias and lymphomas. It may now be applicable for the treatment of severe autoimmune diseases, such as therapy-resistant rheumatoid arthritis and multiple sclerosis. Studies in animal models show that the transfer of haematopoietic stem cells can reverse autoimmunity, and several mechanistic pathways may explain this phenomenon.

A lethal autoimmune disease succumbs to stem cells
https://www.nature.com/articles/d41586-018-00078-6

•	The results are consistent with two previous stem-cell trials, and should help to establish stem-cell transplants as a standard treatment for individuals with severe scleroderma, according to the researchers.

Human Umbilical Cord Blood Stem Cells Infusion in Spinal Cord Injury: Engraftment and Beneficial Influence on Behavior

https://www.liebertpub.com/doi/abs/10.1089/152581603322023007

- Open-field test scores of spinal cord injured rats treated with human cord blood at 5 days were significantly improved as compared to scores of rats similarly injured but treated at day 1 as well as the otherwise untreated injured group. The results suggest that cord blood stem cells are beneficial in reversing the behavioral effects of spinal cord injury, even when infused 5 days after injury. Human cord blood-derived cells were observed in injured areas, but not in non-injured areas, of rat spinal cords, and were never seen in corresponding areas of spinal cord of non-injured animals. The results are consistent with the hypothesis that cord blood-derived stem cells migrate to and participate in the healing of neurological defects caused by traumatic assault.

Bone Marrow Mononuclear Cells Have Neurovascular Tropism and Improve Diabetic Neuropathy

https://stemcellsjournals.onlinelibrary.wiley.com/doi/full/10.1002/stem.87

• In this study, we showed that the transplantation of BMNCs restored the vascularity and function of diabetic nerves, supporting the hypothesis that neural vascularity is pathophysiologically associated with the development and reversal of DN

Multipotent Stem Cells from Umbilical Cord: Cord Is Richer than Blood!

https://stemcellsjournals.onlinelibrary.wiley.com/doi/10.1634/stemcells.2007-0381

• Despite the advantages of HSC from UCB in hematopoietic reconstitution [13, 14–15], results from the present study demonstrated that UC, and not UCB, is the best choice for isolating MSCs for future applications. Until very recently, BM has been considered the main source of MSCs. Panepucci et al. demonstrated that MSCs derived from UC and BM are highly similar at the transcriptional level, reinforcing the usefulness of UC from neonates.

Life-Sparing Effect of Human Cord Blood-Mesenchymal Stem Cells in Experimental Acute Kidney Injury†

https://stemcellsjournals.onlinelibrary.wiley.com/doi/10.1002/stem.293

- CONCLUSION In conclusion, in a murine model of AKI, hCB-MSC treatment promotes kidney regeneration and prolongs survival better than any other cellular approach attempted so far. These effects appear to be mediated by a paracrine action of hCB-MSCs on tubular cells involving lowering oxidative stress, apoptosis, and inflammation. These data indicate that hCB-MSCs have to be considered as one possible future option for cellular therapy of AKI in humans.

Human Umbilical Cord-Derived Mesenchymal Stromal Cells Improve Left Ventricular Function, Perfusion, and Remodeling in a Porcine Model of Chronic Myocardial Ischemia

https://stemcellsjournals.onlinelibrary.wiley.com/doi/10.5966/sctm.2015-0298

- Conclusion This is the first study to provide evidence that intracoronary delivery combined with multiple intravenous infusions of UC-MSCs improves LV function, perfusion, and remodeling in a large animal model of chronic myocardial ischemia. In the present study, we observed neither tumor nor teratoma formation in human UC-MSC-transplanted animals, and no sustained ventricular arrhythmia or anaphylaxis was observed. Because these cells can be isolated from medical waste, expanded, banked, and administered to patients at any time without immunological rejection, human UC-MSCs might be an ideal cell source for cardiac cell therapy and hold promise as an off-the-shelf product.

Intravenous Infusion of Umbilical Cord Blood-Derived Mesenchymal Stem Cells in Rheumatoid Arthritis: A Phase Ia Clinical Trial

https://stemcellsjournals.onlinelibrary.wiley.com/doi/10.1002/sctm.18-0031

- Conclusion This is the first phase Ia study of RA patients that evaluated the safety and tolerability of a single intravenous infusion with hUCB-MSCs and with cell numbers of up to 1×10^8, revealing an acceptable safety profile. Conclusions regarding efficacy in phase I trials are limited, and although evaluation of disease activity was not the primary objective of this study, a single infusion of hUCB-MSCs effectively reduced the mean DAS28 at week 4. Considering favorable safety profiles, intravenous infusion of hUCB-MSCs may constitute a therapeutic option for patients with RA, who are refractory to or intolerant of

MTX. There is a wide array of opportunities for future clinical studies with different hUCB-MSC infusion strategies in which safety profiles should be carefully monitored and outcome measures further refined for optimized effectiveness evaluations.

Therapeutic potential of allogeneic mesenchymal stromal cells transplantation for lupus nephritis.

https://www.ncbi.nlm.nih.gov/pubmed/30290717

- Proteinuria levels improved dramatically during the 1st month after treatment and the ameliorations were sustained throughout the follow-up period. SLEDAI scores revealed early, durable, and substantial remissions that were complete for two patients and partial for the third patient and that permitted medication doses to be reduced 50-90%. These favourable outcomes support completion of the randomized and controlled MSC trial for SLE.

Mesenchymal Stromal Cells Based Therapy in Systemic Sclerosis: Rational and Challenges

https://www.ncbi.nlm.nih.gov/pmc/articles/PMC6146027/

- The ability of MSCs to positively influence processes such as immunosuppression, angiogenesis and inflammation generated a lot of interest and enthusiasm from clinicians and researchers alike. It is apparent that many questions remain unanswered, however what is becoming clear is that MSCs-based therapy should considered as a safe and potentially efficient therapeutic option in the management of advanced stage of SSc.

The Use of Human Mesenchymal Stem Cells as Therapeutic Agents for the in vivo Treatment of Immune-Related Diseases: A Systematic Review

https://www.ncbi.nlm.nih.gov/pmc/articles/PMC6141714/

- In this systematic review, the treatment of many types of immune-related diseases was conducted through the administration of hMSCs. Positive results were usually reported and attributed to the paracrine effects of molecules secreted by hMSCs on immune cells. In conclusion, despite the need for further studies, the treatment of immune-related diseases through the administration of hMSCs is progressively ceasing being only a promising possibility and becoming a reality.

Mesenchymal stem cells alleviate experimental autoimmune cholangitis through immunosuppression and cytoprotective function mediated by galectin-9

https://www.ncbi.nlm.nih.gov/pmc/articles/PMC6142687/

- In summary, the present study shows that UC-MSCs exert profound inhibitory effects on inflammatory responses to alleviate liver injury in experimental autoimmune cholangitis mice. Furthermore, UC-MSCs inhibit Th1 and Th17 cell responses as well as aberrant chemokine activities through Gal-9–mediated immunosuppression. Additionally, the induction of Gal-9 in UC-MSCs is mediated by the STAT and JNK signaling pathways. Our results provide novel insights into the clinical application of UC-MSCs in the treatment of PBC.

The Beneficial Effect of Human Amnion Mesenchymal Cells in Inhibition of Inflammation and Induction of Neuronal Repair in EAE Mice

https://www.ncbi.nlm.nih.gov/pmc/articles/PMC6035808/

- Recently, accumulating evidence showed that MSCs from different origins, including adipose-derived, bone marrow-derived, and umbilical cord-derived, could attenuate the disease progression in EAE animal models [27–29]. Furthermore, autologous bone marrow-derived MSCs transplantation and allogeneic umbilical cord-derived MSCs transplantation for the treatment of MS have been proved safe and effective in clinical trials, which showed that treatment improved the course of the disease, reduced the inflammatory response, and promoted neuroprotection

TGF-β and mesenchymal stromal cells in regenerative medicine, autoimmunity and cancer.

https://www.ncbi.nlm.nih.gov/pubmed/29954665

•	Multipotent mesenchymal stromal cells (MSCs) represent a promising cell-based therapy in regenerative medicine and for the treatment of inflammatory/autoimmune diseases. Importantly, MSCs have emerged as an important contributor to the tumor stroma with both pro- and anti-tumorigenic effects

Modulation of autophagy as new approach in mesenchymal stem cell-based therapy.

https://www.ncbi.nlm.nih.gov/pubmed/29787987

•	Here, we review the current literature describing mechanisms by which modulation of autophagy strengthens pro-angiogenic and immunosuppressive characteristics of MSCs in animal models of multiple sclerosis, osteoporosis, diabetic limb ischemia, myocardial infarction, acute graft-versus-host disease, kidney and liver diseases. Obtained results suggest that modulation of autophagy in MSCs may represent a new therapeutic approach that could enhance efficacy of MSCs in the treatment of ischemic and autoimmune diseases.

Therapeutic Applications of Mesenchymal Stem Cells for Systemic Lupus Erythematosus.

https://www.ncbi.nlm.nih.gov/pubmed/29767288

- Mesenchymal stem cells (MSCs) have been intensively studied and applied in regenerative medicine and tissue engineering. Recently, their immune modulation functions make them as attractive potential approaches for autoimmune disease treatment. Systemic lupus erythematosus (SLE) is one type of chronic autoimmune diseases with multi-organ damaged by the immune system. Although current available treatments are effective for some patients, others are refractory for these therapies. The immuno-modulatory and regenerative characteristics of MSCs make them as one promising candidate for treating SLE.

Cell therapies for refractory rheumatoid arthritis.

https://www.ncbi.nlm.nih.gov/pubmed/29745893

- Recently, cell-based therapies have become the focus, attracting more attention due to their potential for remission induction. Several immune-regulatory cell types, such as haematopoietic stem cells, mesenchymal stem cells and regulatory T cells have been defined as novel targets.

Mesenchymal stem cell transplantation in systemic lupus erythematous, a mesenchymal stem cell disorder.

https://www.ncbi.nlm.nih.gov/pubmed/29631514

- MSCs from SLE patients have demonstrated defects such as aberrant cytokine production. Moreover, impaired phenotype, growth and immunomodulatory functions of MSCs from patients with SLE in comparison to healthy controls have been reported. Therefore, it is hypothesized that SLE is potentially an MSC-mediated disease and, as a result, allogeneic rather than autologous MSC transplantation can be argued to be a potentially advantageous therapy for patients with SLE.

Hematopoietic and mesenchymal stem cell transplantation for severe and refractory systemic lupus erythematosus.

https://www.ncbi.nlm.nih.gov/pubmed/23770628

- Recently, growing evidence suggests that the functions of hematopoietic stem cells (HSCs) and mesenchymal stem cells (MSCs) are disrupted in SLE pathology. And HSC or MSC transplantation

(HSCT/MSCT) can offer an effective and safe therapy for the severe SLE patients, resulting in disease clinical remission and improvement of organ dysfunction.

The protective effects of human umbilical cord mesenchymal stem cells on damaged ovarian function: A comparative study.

https://www.ncbi.nlm.nih.gov/pubmed/27464625

- A higher level of expression of anti-apoptotic and antioxidant enzymes was noted in the ovaries of groups treated with hUCMSCs. These parameters were enhanced more when mice were treated with hUCMSCs for 1 month than when they treated with hUCMSCs for 2 weeks. IV was better able to restore ovarian function than MI. These results suggest that both methods of transplantation may improve ovarian function and that IV transplantation of hUCMSCs can significantly improve ovarian function and structural parameters more than MI transplantation of hUCMSCs can. Human umbilical cord mesenchymal stem cells improve the reserve function of perimenopausal ovary via a paracrine mechanism.

https://www.ncbi.nlm.nih.gov/pubmed/28279229

- CONCLUSIONS: Our results suggest that hUCMSCs can promote ovarian expression of HGF, VEGF, and IGF-1 through secreting those cytokines, resulting in improving ovarian reserve function and withstanding ovarian senescence.

Intramuscular injection of human umbilical cord-derived mesenchymal stem cells improves cardiac function in dilated cardiomyopathy rats

https://www.ncbi.nlm.nih.gov/pmc/articles/PMC5273808/

- BACKGROUND: Stem cells provide a promising candidate for the treatment of the fatal pediatric dilated cardiomyopathy (DCM). This study aimed to investigate the effects of intramuscular injection of human umbilical cord-derived mesenchymal stem cells (hUCMSCs) on the cardiac function of a DCM rat model.

- CONCLUSIONS: Intramuscular injection of UCMSCs can improve DCM-induced cardiac function impairment and protect the myocardium. These effects may be mediated by regulation of relevant cytokines in serum and the myocardium.

Long term effect and safety of Wharton's jelly-derived mesenchymal stem cells on type 2 diabetes

https://www.ncbi.nlm.nih.gov/pmc/articles/PMC4997981/

- In conclusion, the findings of the present study suggested that WJ-MSC infusion may effectively ameliorate hyperglycemia, improve islet β-cell function and reduce the incidence of diabetic complications over a sustained period of time. Despite the fact that WJ-MSC infusion does not appear to attenuate insulin resistance, WJ-MSC infusion may have therapeutic potential as a novel agent for the treatment of T2DM.

Long term effect and safety of Wharton's jelly-derived mesenchymal stem cells on type 2 diabetes

https://www.researchgate.net/publication/305677302_Long _term_effect_and_safety_of_Wharton's_jelly- derived_mesenchymal_stem_cells_on_type_2_diabetes

- Cellular therapies offer novel opportunities for the treatment of type 2 diabetes mellitus (T2DM). The present study evaluated the long-term efficacy and safety of infusion of Wharton's jelly-derived mesenchymal stem cells (WJ-MSC) on T2DM. A total of 61 patients with T2DM were randomly divided into two groups on the basis of basal therapy; patients in group I were administered WJ-MSC intravenous infusion twice, with a four-week interval, and patients in group II were treated with normal saline as control. During the 36-month follow-up period, the occurrence of any adverse effects and the results of clinical and laboratory examinations were recorded and evaluated. The lack of acute or chronic adverse effects in group I was consistent with group II.. Blood glucose, glycosylated hemoglobin, C-peptide, homeostasis model assessment of pancreatic islet β-cell function and incidence of diabetic complications in group I were significantly improved, as compared with group II during the 36-month follow-up. The results of the present study demonstrated that infusion of WJ-MSC improved the function of islet β-cells and reduced the incidence of diabetic complications, although the precise mechanisms are yet to be elucidated. The infusion of WJ-MSC may be an effective option for the treatment of patients with type 2 diabetes.

Mesenchymal stem cells in tissue repair.
https://www.ncbi.nlm.nih.gov/pubmed/24027567

• Mesenchymal stem cells have become a major focus for a potential resource in therapeutic cell-based therapies. MSCs are multipotent cells derived from stromal tissue, which have the capacity to differentiate into mesodermal and endodermal types of cells. Not only do MSCs have the capacity to differentiate into different types of cells depending on the tissue matrix, they also actively contribute to their milieu by secreting soluble products that actively participate in MSC and surrounding cell phenotype.

Mesenchymal stem cells from human umbilical cord express preferentially secreted factors related to neuroprotection, neurogenesis, and angiogenesis.
https://www.ncbi.nlm.nih.gov/pubmed/23991127
- Our results confirmed that WJ-MSCs secreted highly levels of CXCL5 compared with BM-MSCs.

Therapeutic potential of human umbilical cord mesenchymal stem cells in the treatment of rheumatoid arthritis.
https://www.ncbi.nlm.nih.gov/pubmed/21080925
- In conclusion, human UC-MSCs suppressed the various inflammatory effects of FLSs and T cells of RA in vitro, and attenuated the development of CIA in vivo, strongly suggesting that UC-MSCs might be a therapeutic strategy in RA. In addition, the immunosuppressive activitiy of UC-MSCs could be prolonged by the participation of Tregs.

Stem cell delivery of therapies for brain disorders
https://www.ncbi.nlm.nih.gov/pmc/articles/PMC4106911/

- MSCs have the potential as cellular vehicles for drugs and other molecules to treat patients with neural diseases such as GBM, AD, PD, TBI and other neuropathologies for which limited treatment options exist. When considering the limitations of current methods of drug delivery to the brain, MSCs have the potential to become a safe cellular delivery vehicle containing a prodrug as well as ectopically expressed genes for targeted delivery. The affinity for MSCs to migrate to the brain combined with the relative ease for expanded MSCs make them attractive for gene and drug delivery.

www.ingramcontent.com/pod-product-compliance
Lightning Source LLC
Chambersburg PA
CBHW071410210526
45465CB00001B/321